The Power of Guilt

Dr. Chris Moore is a professor of psychology and former dean of science at Dalhousie University in Canada, as well as a former Canada Research Chair at the University of Toronto. He has spent his career studying human social understanding and relations, and has published over 100 research papers, edited 5 books and special issues of academic journals, and authored *The Development of Commonsense Psychology* (Psychology Press, 2006). Moore's work has been cited in mainstream print publications such as *Psychology Today*, *Today's Parent*, and the *New York Times*.

THE
POWER
OF
GUILT

Chris Moore Ph.D

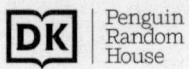

First published in the United States in 2025 by Collins, an imprint of HarperCollins Publishers Ltd

This edition published in the United Kingdom in 2026 by

August Books, an imprint of
Canelo Digital Publishing Limited,
20 Vauxhall Bridge Road,
London SW1V 2SA
United Kingdom

A Penguin Random House Company
The authorised representative in the EEA is Dorling Kindersley Verlag GmbH. Arnulfstr. 124, 80636 Munich, Germany

Copyright © Chris Moore 2025

The moral right of Chris Moore to be identified as the creator of this work has been asserted in accordance with the Copyright, Designs and Patents Act, 1988.

All rights reserved. No part of this publication may be reproduced or transmitted in any form or by any means, electronic or mechanical, including photocopy, recording, or any information storage and retrieval system, without permission in writing from the publisher.

No part of this book may be used or reproduced in any manner for the purpose of training artificial intelligence technologies or systems. In accordance with Article 4(3) of the DSM Directive 2019/790, Canelo expressly reserves this work from the text and data mining exception.

A CIP catalogue record for this book is available from the British Library.

Ebook ISBN 978 1 83598 412 3
Hardback ISBN 978 1 83598 409 3
Trade Paperback ISBN 978 1 83598 511 3

Printed and bound in Great Britain by Clays Ltd, Elcograf S.p.A.

Look for more great books at
www.augustbooks.co | www.dk.com

For the victims of the accident.

You showed me the power of guilt and forgiveness.

Table of Contents

Introduction: *A Personal Experience of Guilt*   1

Part I: *The Nature of Guilt*

Chapter One: *What Is Guilt?*   15

Chapter Two: *What Is Guilt For?*   31

Chapter Three: *The Development of Guilt and Conscience in Children*   50

Chapter Four: *Guilt-Proneness*   76

Part II: *Guilt in Everyday Life*

Chapter Five: *Guilt in Adult Relationships*   101

Chapter Six: *Parental Guilt*   126

Chapter Seven: *Guilt and Adult Children*   147

Chapter Eight: *Guilt Gone Awry*   165

Part III: *Guilt in Society*

Chapter Nine: *Guilt in Religion*   193

Chapter Ten: *Guilt in the Law*   214

Chapter Eleven: *Collective Guilt*   238

Conclusion: *Making Friends with Guilt*   269

Acknowledgments   275

Notes   277

Introduction

A Personal Experience of Guilt

When I was twenty, after finishing exams at the end of my second year at university, I attended a house party a little way out of town. It was a warm, late-spring evening, and the exuberance of the end of the year was rampant among the partygoers. I was feeling exhilarated—I had completed my final psychology exam of the year, and after beginning my university career with considerable uncertainty about my career path, had discovered my true intellectual passion, a passion that remains with me even now, over forty years later.

Late into the evening, after too many drinks, I was standing in the driveway with three friends, all of us equally intoxicated. The party was still in full swing, but we were ready to call it a night. We noticed a car in the driveway with the keys in the ignition. One of us—I do not remember whom—suggested we get in and drive back to college. It was a fair distance back, there were no buses, and we certainly couldn't walk. How else were we to get home? I took the seat on the front passenger side and promptly fell asleep. The next thing I remember, I was sitting by the side of the road, with blood on my face and the flashing lights of police and ambulance vehicles all around.

Evidently, we had gotten into an accident, and I had hit the windshield, which shattered, lacerating my forehead. My friends were talking to the police, but I was loaded into an ambulance and taken to the hospital for emergency surgery. I remember nothing more about that night. It was only after I awoke from surgery early the next morning that I learned what had happened. We had hit a group of fellow students cycling the same road back to town. Some of them had been injured and one had been killed.

I spent the next week in the hospital, in a bed on the plastic surgery ward, as my head healed. It was a traditional hospital ward with perhaps a dozen beds, most of which were occupied by patients requiring skin grafts. I was there because the damage to my forehead was quite extensive and the surgeon's team had explored the possibility of skin grafts to complete the work, but fortunately, they managed to stitch the wound in a patchwork that would allow much faster healing. It would also leave me with a scar reminding me of the accident for the rest of my life.

On the ward, I was nervous to engage with my fellow in-patients, afraid that they would be aware of the reasons for my confinement. I lay in bed with little to do but reflect on what had happened and what I had done. My memory of the events of that night was patchy—not surprising given my intoxication and the injury I had sustained. But the facts were clear, and they were devastating. Even though societal attitudes toward drunk driving were not nearly as condemning then as they are today, I had taken a car that did not belong to me, enabled a friend to drive while drunk, and thereby participated in a chain of events that led to the death of a fellow student, as well as injuries to others.

When something so drastic happens, it is natural for our thoughts to go first to the people in our lives who are affected. In my case, the list was long. I thought first of my family. My relationship with my parents was sometimes strained. And now I had been irresponsible in a completely unprecedented and damaging way. I had disrupted their carefully constructed middle-class Catholic family existence. How would I cope with their inevitable rejection? I thought of my friends in the accident with me. How could we look at each other again? Why had we participated in this rash and endangering action? Had I encouraged the others, who might have otherwise stepped away? I thought of the injured students and, in particular, the one who had died. I did not know them, but they were my peers, just starting out in their adult lives. I might easily have been in their place, but instead, I was responsible for derailing their journeys and, in one tragic case, terminating it. It was difficult to contemplate a more damaging act. Entwined with all these thoughts was my concern about the implications for me. Had I, in one act of reckless impulsivity, ruined my chosen career path? Given all of this, how could I live with myself knowing that my actions had cost someone his life?

Introduction

As these thoughts tumbled over each other in those first hours after learning the awful truth of that night, I fell into a morass of guilt, shame, remorse, and fear. At the time, I could hardly parse these emotions; I was simply stunned by their intensity.

As the week passed, my agonizing was punctuated by visitors. Remarkably, with each visit, I felt a bit better. It was as if each visitor added a length of rope to pull me out of the deep pit of my misery. Even then, I was struck by how the kindness of my visitors worked to counteract the negativity of my mental state. As I recall that time now, I see that it was the reconciliation offered by these visitors that effected my recovery from my emotional desperation.

Two visits stand out in my memory even now. First, my parents made the long drive from our hometown immediately. They appeared at my bedside the day after my surgery. Both were dressed neatly, which was consistent with their carefully nurtured middle-class style. Normally, they would be restrained in public, but that day, their emotion was clear on their faces as they approached my bed. There was a softness in their demeanor that was unfamiliar to me. They told me that yes, I had done an extraordinarily stupid and harmful thing, but nevertheless, they still loved me and had faith in me. These were not the kind of words that, with their stoic British reserve, my parents were known for. I listened to them with my head bowed; I could not look at them in that moment. It took a minute for their words to sink in. I remember well thinking at the time that this was the first occasion in my life that they had talked to me in this way. It had taken an extremely regrettable act to provoke a reaction from them that allowed me to feel truly, unconditionally loved by them. I realized then that without really knowing it, I had, up to that point, believed that my parents' love for me depended on my being good, or obedient, or successful in school. Their visit was critical, not just for revealing to me that my parents loved me, but for dissipating my shame. I was not a bad person; I had just acted stupidly.

The second significant visit was from friends of the student who had died. I do not remember exactly how many came, but one of them had been in the group of cyclists we had hit, and others were part of their circle of friends. I did not know them at all and was shocked to see them. I had no resources to handle this situation and lay in my hospital bed, dumbstruck as they stood around me. It turned out they were members of the Christian Union, for whom a life of forgiveness was fundamental. They had come to let me know that they forgave me and held no ill feelings toward me. Furthermore, they assured me that the student who had died and his family would hold no hard feelings toward me. For them, these events were inevitably part of God's plan. Only God could judge; their responsibility was to love and serve Him.

By that time in my life, I had renounced the Christianity of my own upbringing, but I knew the significance of forgiveness to leading a virtuous Christian life. It is difficult to overestimate the impact this visit had on me. Even now, thinking about it decades later and reliving that moment, my eyes well up. What I remember clearly is that with this visit, incredibly, the intense guilt I felt began to dissolve.

After a week in the hospital, my head had healed enough for me to be discharged into the hands of the police. As I sat in the back of the squad car, the two officers in front berated me with their opinions of my character. They asked me how I could live with myself. Quite reasonably, they viewed me as an entitled and privileged student with no sense of responsibility, who deserved to be severely punished. But their verbal assault washed over me. I remember looking at the backs of their heads and thinking, *Who are you to rebuke me in this way when the people who were harmed have already forgiven me?* I knew I had broken the law and I deserved to be punished for what I had done, but I also knew my real mistake was to get so drunk that I lost all sense of responsibility and control. At that moment, I *knew* I was guilty of the crime of unlawfully taking a car, but I did not really *feel* guilty about it.

I was taken to the local police station and charged with what, in the circumstances, seemed like a rather minor crime: "taking and driving away," a lesser form of automobile theft, as there was no intent on our part to keep the car. Only my friend who had driven the car and directly caused the accident was charged with the more serious crime of "causing death by dangerous driving." I was released on bail and ordered to appear in court at a later date. I went back to my parents' house for the summer and, after hearing from my college that I had been suspended for a year, prepared to take that year to work and try to get my life back on track.

The trial was scheduled for three months after the accident. My lawyer prepared carefully for the hearing. He assured me that for a first-time offender on a relatively minor charge, I would receive a fine and likely some form of community service. In court, I sat next to my three friends as we listened to the prosecution recount the events of that night. We could not help but be profoundly remorseful. Like the others, I pled guilty to the charge and apologized to the court for my action. The judge was unimpressed. My lawyer was as shocked as I was when the judge announced a sentence of six months in prison for me and my two friends who were also passengers. Our friend who had driven the car received a sentence of nine months in prison, a relatively lenient sentence for his crime. In his remarks, the judge argued that, despite the different charges, in his view we were all similarly responsible for the terrible outcome, and he was reluctant to differentiate significantly among us in the punishment meted out.

After sentencing, I was immediately taken into custody and spent the next week in a holding cell in a high-security prison before being transferred to an open prison to serve out my time reading and playing cards with white-collar criminals. To be perfectly honest, there was a part of me that was grateful for that time. Although the intense guilt I had felt in the immediate aftermath of the accident had been largely dissipated by my hospital visitors, I was responsible for the events of that night, and I needed to accept a suitable punishment. At the time, a prison term and a criminal record was the stigma that seemed appropriate. I also could not shake the feeling that, as the judge had suggested, I was almost as responsible for the death of our fellow student as my friend who had driven the car. In fact, I felt guilty that the driver would have to carry the burden of this crime in a way that the rest of us would be spared. To receive an equal punishment as he did felt right.

My lawyer, like those of the other two passengers, did not share this perspective and convinced my parents that my sentence should be appealed. He was sure that the judge had overstepped the mark and should not have punished the passengers so severely. Even if we did share responsibility, the fact was that the crime we had been convicted of was a minor offense, and there was no legal precedent for a punishment as harsh as ours. He also suggested that the judge had responded to implicit pressure to make an example of reckless and dangerous student behavior in a city where town and gown relations could be fraught.

He was right. On appeal, he argued that we had been punished for the severity of the consequences and not for the crime we had committed. The appeal hearing judge agreed, and my sentence, like those of the other two passengers, was reduced to time served—three months. I was immediately released from prison to return home and reflect on a set of experiences I had certainly not anticipated when I set out for university.

During the rest of the year that I was suspended from university, I read broadly in the areas of emotional and personality psychology. I was intent on making a career in psychology, and now I had a new motivation for studying: trying to make sense of my experience. Why had I acted in the way that I did? But even more significantly, why had I responded to learning of the accident as I did and how was it that the reactions of those around me had such an impact on my recovery from the depths of despair I first experienced?

My feelings of guilt grew in the first few hours as I learned of the consequences of my action. But although there was a single action, there was not a single source of guilt. I felt guilt in relation to my parents, to my friends, and to the victims of our crime. These manifestations of guilt were quite independent, and they reflected the different ways I related to these different people. I felt guilt in relation to my parents because I had let them down, failed to meet their expectations and, indeed, any reasonable standard of a dutiful son. I felt guilt in relation to my friends because I could not dismiss the possibility that I was in part responsible for the circumstances that befell them as well as me. I felt the most intense guilt in relation to the victims, because they were the ones most directly and dramatically harmed. Overall, it was clear that my action had different repercussions for different relationships, and a different manifestation of guilt was attached to each.

Although difficult to articulate, the emotional flavor of these diverse forms of guilt also seemed different. With my friends, with whom I had essentially symmetrical relationships as peers, my guilt was more a sense of uneasiness that our friendships were threatened by what had happened. I searched my memory for a record of the conversation that led us to take the car, but it was blank. What if it had been my suggestion initially? If, as I worried, I had been more of a leader than a follower in the decision to take the car that night, then I had greater responsibility and I needed to find a way to make things right with them. This guilt was the least intense of them all, and it appeared even then to have a clear and obvious motivating purpose: to heal any possible harm to our friendships.

Introduction

My relationship with my parents, naturally, was very different from my relationship with my friends. Even when we are adults, our relationships with our parents are colored by the long history of obedience and subordination to them. We look to our parents for love, guidance, and direction, and we generally want to please them. The guilt in relation to my parents weighed more heavily on my sense of self and was more akin to shame—my action had revealed me to be a bad person. I say *revealed* because I did not think that my action *made* me a bad person. Rather, I believed I was *already* a bad person and this action had demonstrated that fact to my parents and to the world. This shame made me feel depressed and helpless.

Even though I did not know the victims of the accident, the guilt I felt in relation to them was a much more powerful, existential guilt, consonant with the extent of the harm caused, that left me feeling that a seismic shift had occurred in my life. That guilt encompassed both the hurt I had caused to the victims and their families and the repercussions for my own life. I could not imagine at that time how it would ever be possible to escape from under the oppressive weight of that remorse. I knew that everything was changed for me that night and there was no way back to the life that I had had before.

Of course, I was also guilty of a crime. This guilt seemed at the time—and still now seems—of a very different kind. I fully accepted that I was guilty of the crime I was charged with, but I also knew that my recklessness with alcohol was the real culprit, and so I did not really *feel* guilty about taking the car.

The legal case, and the way the judge attempted to treat the four of us similarly even though we were charged with crimes of different severity, brought home to me the fact that ours was really a group crime, and as such we shared the guilt. Would any of us have taken the car that night if we had been on our own? I think it is very unlikely. We were all conscientious, law-abiding youths. Alone, our standards for responsible behavior would have prevented such an event. But together, a different, group mentality kicked in. We encouraged each other, testing our own ability to be reckless against that of the others. The crime was a result of the group of the four of us acting together, acting in a way that none of us would have alone. If the action depended on the existence of our group, then it makes sense to say that *the group* was responsible, and *the group* was collectively guilty. That is why the judge felt he could reasonably require a similar level of punishment for all of us. But the law is not designed to manage collective guilt. It is individuals who are charged with crimes and individuals who are punished, and so the legal appropriateness of his sentencing was dismissed on appeal.

Understanding these different forms of guilt is not complete without also understanding the ways in which they are resolved. I consider myself to be almost unbelievably fortunate that they were all addressed in such a short space of time for me. It could so easily have been otherwise. I was lucky to have parents who, although they rarely showed it in everyday life and often came across as judgmental, were able to express their unconditional love for me when it was most needed. Not long after I got out of the hospital, I was able to get together with my friends, and we shared apologies and committed to a completely joint responsibility for what we had done. I still marvel to this day that some of the innocent victims of our gross irresponsibility came to my bedside and explicitly forgave me for my action, absolving me. Finally, my guilt over breaking the law was dealt with through the workings of the legal system. Within a year, having plumbed the depths of despair in the immediate aftermath of the accident, I had been pulled through the emotional and legal repercussions of the episode and had come out the other side.

In the years since, I have imagined what might have happened if I had not been so lucky. What if my parents had judged me harshly, punished me in some way, and continued to hold this action against me for dishonoring them or my family? Would this evaluation have contributed to the shame of a negative self-image weighing me down throughout my life? Imagine if one of my friends had also died in the accident while I survived. Would I have been plagued by "survivor guilt"—the guilt that can arise in people who have been exposed to or witnessed death and stayed alive—whenever I thought about those events? And most troubling, the victims or their families might not have been committed Christians who prioritized forgiveness as a core value, and might never have forgiven us. It is interesting to me that the imagination of these alternative outcomes leads me even now to genuinely experience, although in a somewhat attenuated way, feelings of guilt. Under any of these circumstances, it is very likely that I would still be dealing with significant guilt today. These speculations have convinced me that a healthy recovery from guilt is fundamentally dependent on forgiveness by and reconciliation with those whom one has harmed. When forgiveness and reconciliation do not happen, guilt will fester.

Forgiveness and reconciliation usually have to be earned. Again, I was fortunate that they were offered to me without me having to work for them or show I deserved them. My parents and the students who visited me in the hospital spontaneously offered their forgiveness. My friends and I were all in the same position; none of us bore any greater responsibility than the others, and the shared experience, if anything, brought us closer together in the immediate aftermath. My wider circle of friends were all equally spontaneously compassionate— in no case was there judgment; instead, there was sympathy and support. Only in the case of my legal guilt did I have to earn society's forgiveness by taking my punishment. The prison sentence I received was supposed to serve that function. (And although my legal guilt was resolved by serving my prison sentence, I do believe that for this kind of crime, incarceration is poorly suited to genuine reconciliation, and perhaps a form of community service would have been more meaningful.)

This episode in my early adulthood taught me an enormous amount about guilt and the role it played in my own experience. Perhaps my most fundamental takeaway was that guilt is not simply the result of doing something wrong, whatever that may mean. Rather, guilt arises from doing something that has damaged a social relationship. Of course, hurting a social relationship often overlaps with what is considered wrong by society, but it is the damage to the relationship that is critical to the experience of guilt. That is why I felt guilt in different ways— through a single act, I had caused damage to different relationships.

This idea stands in contrast to the typical dictionary definitions of guilt. If you look up *guilt* in dictionaries, you will generally find two kinds. For example, the *Cambridge Dictionary* defines guilt as "a *feeling* of worry or unhappiness that you have because you have done something wrong, such as causing harm to another person," or "the *fact* of having done something wrong or committed a crime."[1] Other standard dictionaries make the same distinction. The first definition focuses on guilt as a negative feeling in connection with having done something wrong. The second definition equates guilt as the state of transgression of a rule imposed by some authority. The first treats guilt as a subjective or psychological experience; the second as an objective fact.

How do these two meanings of guilt—the subjective and the objective—manage to live side by side? Both meanings cast guilt primarily as the result of wrongdoing. But the subjective definition focuses on *why* we care about guilt—because it is a negative emotional experience. It does not really help us understand what we feel guilty about or what counts as wrongdoing. The objective definition tells us whether we *are* guilty, but it doesn't tell us why we should care.

The traditional approach to the reconciliation of these two meanings of guilt is that the objective meaning came first and the subjective meaning was derived from it. This approach is consistent with the etymology of the word *guilt*, which originates in English from the Old English word *gylt*, meaning "crime" or "debt."[2] According to this view, moral—and subsequently legal—rules were passed down from authority (God, the king, lawmakers, etc.) and were to be obeyed under threat of punishment. Transgression of such rules resulted in objective guilt and consequently punishment. Inevitably, the breaking of such rules, or even the thought of breaking the rules, led to feelings of distress or concern, and these feelings came to be known as subjective guilt. These days, it is common for *guilt* to be defined as a "moral emotion." For example, Wikipedia presently defines *guilt* as "a moral emotion that occurs when a person believes or realizes—accurately or not—that they have compromised their own standards of conduct or have violated universal moral standards and bear significant responsibility for that violation."[3] This definition explicitly links the feeling of guilt with the fact of moral rule violation.

Nevertheless, it is clear that the two kinds of guilt may exist quite easily in isolation from each other. Someone may feel guilty about an action without it involving the explicit transgression of any moral rule. (I feel guilty that I spend more time working than my wife would like me to.) And one may be guilty of acting illegally with no experience of guilt. (I'm happy to jaywalk if it will get me to where I'm going faster.) This loose association between the subjective and the objective forms of guilt points to something missing from our understanding of guilt.

To my mind, this standard approach to understanding guilt misses a critical piece of the picture: why certain kinds of actions are deemed wrong by moral or legal authorities in the first place. In fact, almost all acts of wrongdoing are ones that harm other people with whom we have some form of social relationship. Rather than interpret guilt in terms of wrongdoing, we need to begin our understanding of guilt by considering its role in managing our social relationships. We must think of guilt as primarily an interpersonal phenomenon. What I mean by this is that guilt is something that occurs in the context of relationships *between* people rather than simply *within* a person or with reference to a set of rules.[4] That's not to say we do not *feel* guilt "inside us." Guilt is a real emotional experience. However, the experience of guilt is fundamentally tied to the ways in which we interact with other people. In the simplest terms, guilt arises when a person perceives that their relationship with another person has been damaged in some way. Most guilt follows from doing something that harms the other person in the relationship. But, sometimes guilt can arise even when we did nothing to cause harm. Perhaps we feel guilty that we got a promotion when our colleague and friend did not. The fact that guilt can arise in situations where we have little or no direct responsibility for a challenge to a relationship tells us that it is the threat to the relationship that is central to the experience of guilt. Guilt is the emotional signal that tells us we should attempt to repair this damage. That is why it is relieved by forgiveness—forgiveness by the other tells us that the relationship has been repaired.

The kind of event that I experienced at twenty can shape a life. Even after more than forty years, the memory of this episode is still quite fresh in my mind, perhaps because I have thought about it so frequently over the years. And just as I can still feel and see in the mirror the physical evidence of the accident on my forehead, the experience has left its mark internally. Looking back now, I can see how the experience at the end of my second year as an undergraduate set me on a path of discovery that leads all the way to this book. Those events and the ways my emotional reaction to learning of the accident was tempered and profoundly redirected by the reactions of those most affected led to an enduring fascination with how relationships are damaged and repaired. As a person, I listen to my feelings of guilt to tell me when I might need to work on my relationships. As an academic psychologist, I have been intrigued by the variety of ways in which guilt manifests in our lives and by how the resolution of guilt is dependent on forgiveness and reconciliation. This book tells the story of guilt, a story that is at the same time complicated—guilt shows up in so many areas of our lives—and simple in that in all cases, guilt is the signal that a relationship has been damaged and needs to be healed. We will see that we need to shed the image of guilt as a negative emotional scourge. Instead, guilt is, at its core, a positive force for healthy relationships.

Part I

The Nature of Guilt

Chapter One

What Is Guilt?

During my enforced absence from university, I immersed myself in reading classic texts in psychology, both to prepare for my return to formal studies the following year and to help me understand my experience of that fateful week. The work that moved me most was the landmark work on guilt by Sigmund Freud, *Civilization and Its Discontents*.[1] In this short book, Freud takes on the challenge of explaining how civilization is possible if, as he believed, the human mind is designed to fulfill fundamentally selfish urges.* Reading the book was in itself a guilty pleasure. By that time, I had already been exposed to enough academic psychology from my first two years at university to know that Freudian theory was off-limits for an aspiring research psychologist like me. No works by Freud were included in my university reading lists, and if his theory came up at all, it was only to disparage it as fundamentally unscientific and representative of exactly the wrong way to do psychology. I wasn't supposed to be wasting my time with Freudian flights of fancy.

In reading Freud, I felt like I was panning for gold. To be honest, *Civilization and Its Discontents* is a bit of a mess,[2] as is a lot of Freud's writing. It is obvious that he had been spared both the constraint and the benefit of a good editor. But in sifting through the rambling

---

* Freud's assumption that individual selfish motives come first was consistent with the way that traditional experimental psychology would later conceptualize social behavior. For example, in the field of social learning theory that was dominant during the middle period of the twentieth century and that evolved from learning theory more generally, the origins of social behavior were explained in terms of how the social environment molded behavior according to reward and punishment.

narrative, you come upon nuggets of such original insight that your way of thinking about the mind can shift profoundly. At the same time, these insights are neither the result of scientific study nor articulated clearly enough to allow direct scientific investigation, and so they are often dismissed by those who require empirical justification. It demonstrated to me why his work at one and the same time has had such a profound effect on the way we now think about the mind *and* so frustrates most academic psychologists.

Freud's simple answer to the question of how civilization is possible is guilt. He argued that guilt arises through the tension between two parts of the mind, the "ego," which is the part that seeks ways to achieve one's personal selfish goals, sometimes aggressively, and the "superego," which imposes constraints on the ego.[3] The superego is the Freudian version of conscience, a concept that was, of course, familiar to me. According to Freud, it achieves its power over the ego by "introjecting" anger, or, in other words, by imposing anger reflexively on the person. This self-directed anger is experienced as the feeling of deserving punishment. Guilt leads us to feel that we should be punished for doing bad things, or even for thinking of doing bad things.

This insight is not that novel; it certainly would be familiar to anyone, like me, with a religious upbringing. In the extreme, religious practice has historically included self-flagellation as a form of penitential practice for one's sins. Indeed, there is modern experimental evidence for it. Psychologist Yoel Inbar and his colleagues found that people who were asked to write about episodes where they felt guilty about something they had done administered more intense electric shocks to themselves than people who were asked to write about episodes where they were neutral or sad.[4] The feeling of guilt does lead us to feel that we deserve punishment.

But Freud went further and asked where the superego or conscience comes from. And this was the part that fascinated me. Freud rejected both the idea of a natural morality—an innate sense of right and wrong—and the idea of a morality that is handed down from God and passed on through authorities such as religious figures. He argued that the origin of right and wrong must come in childhood from forces external to the ego, because what is considered right in a civilized society often conflicts with the ego's natural desires: "Since a person's own feelings would not have led him along this path, he must have had a motive to submitting to this extraneous influence." And then there came the shiniest nugget of all: "Such a motive is easily discovered in his helplessness and his dependence on other people, and *it can best be designated as fear of loss of love.*"[5] To me, this second insight was key—guilt is not simply fear of punishment, rather it has its origins in the fear of relationship loss.

Together, these two insights—guilt as self-directed anger and guilt as fear of loss of love—led Freud to propose two core stages in the development of guilt. The earliest is anxiety over the loss of love because of displeasing one's parents. Initially, children inhibit their "bad" behavior because they are fearful of losing their parents' love. Then, in the second stage, the prospect of punishment by their parents for wrongdoing becomes internalized, or applied to the self by the superego. Freud summed up his story as follows: "Thus, we know of two origins of the sense of guilt: one arising from fear of an authority, and the other, later on, arising from fear of the superego."[6]

One final aspect of Freud's theory is important to emphasize. Freud believed that the interplay between ego and superego often occurs unconsciously, both because it first takes place so early in childhood, somewhat out of the reach of later adult memory, and because the emotions involved may be so stressful that they are actively repressed. In particular, when a child feels angry at being prevented by their parents from doing what they want to do (perhaps they really want to poke that electrical outlet or grab that toy from their baby sister), their inclination may be to lash out. But acting that way risks parental rejection, leading to guilt, and so the anger is bottled up, turned inwards, and not allowed to manifest itself.

There are two impacts of this unconscious guilt. One is that as adults, we have little understanding or even memory of the emotional dynamics that led to the establishment of the superego or conscience. So, in adulthood, we tend to experience our conscience as an integral part of who we are, not as something that was established through our interactions with our parents. In my own life, for as long as I can remember, I have been gripped by intense guilt over not doing well enough in school and not working hard enough (which, given my career choice, means not doing well in school as well!). I used to think that this was just a part of my nature. But, as we shall see in Chapter 3, I have come to realize that this guilt has its origins in the role that school played in my relationship with my mother. The second impact of unconscious guilt is that the repressed emotions may leak out as symptoms of psychopathology. We will revisit this process in more detail in Chapter 8.

True to his mission as an interpreter of the human psyche, in *Civilization and Its Discontents* Freud reframed the feeling of guilt in terms of emotional relations between people and not in terms of actions that are in any objective sense "bad." Equally important, Freud showed that guilt is not a simple emotion. It develops in early childhood from fear over the potential loss of one's parents' love and from anger that becomes self-directed. With this account, there was no need to think of guilt as an inherently moral emotion, a response to transgressing certain universal and innate moral laws; the psychological dynamic between children and their parents was all that was needed. To me as a budding psychologist, Freud's story of guilt made a lot of sense.

But there was one aspect of Freud's theory that did not sit so well with me. As I noted earlier, his belief was that from birth, humans are fundamentally motivated to pursue their individual egoistic or selfish goals and must be trained to be social and civilized. Freud recognized the importance of the child's primary relationship with their parents—it was the threat of loss of parental love that initiated the development of the superego. But, once in place, the superego did the rest. For Freud, caring for others is derivative; it comes from a necessary redirection of the ego's fulfillment. According to his view, guilt generated by the superego is the emotional whip that keeps humans socialized.

This way of thinking about guilt did not resonate with me. The intensive immersion in guilt and its resolution that I had experienced during that week in hospital had convinced me that my guilt was first and foremost an emotional response to failing others, with whom I mostly had personal relationships. Once the relationships with those others were healed through their forgiveness, the guilt dissipated, even though the violation of my conscience remained. It seemed to me that anxiety over damaged relationships was the primary motive behind guilt. Freud was likely right that fear over the loss of parental love was the initial cause of guilt in childhood, and I certainly felt this guilt in connection to imagining how my parents would respond to what I had done. However, his fixation on child-parent emotional dynamics had blinded him to a more general truth: guilt arises when we worry that we have harmed our relationships with others, including, but not only, our parents.

The general concern we have for healthy relationships seemed so fundamental to me that I was skeptical of the Freudian view that we start out selfish and must be trained to be social. What if this traditional direction of explanation was backwards? What if the urge to be social—to engage with others, to care for others—comes first, and one's personal motivations stem in large part from a more basic desire to enter into relationships? And what if healthy social interactions and relationships provide the foundation on which the rest of human psychology is built? This way of thinking made more sense to me, and it was the approach to psychology that I became intent on pursuing.

In the early 1980s, when I returned to my studies in psychology, guilt was a topic that was considered hardly at all in academic psychology. Following the contributions of Freud, and the psychoanalysts influenced by him, it fell largely within clinical research and, as such, remained essentially off-limits to academic psychology. In 1981, I began my own research career when I entered the PhD program at the University of Cambridge. For my PhD research, I happened to be working with an advisor whose primary research interest was in young children's cognitive development—the study of how concepts of the physical world develop in early childhood. So, I began to think about how the understanding of the physical world could grow out of social interactions. I was intrigued by the idea that human psychology is deeply constituted through social interactions and relationships. What I mean by this is that our thoughts, desires, and feelings are intricately entwined with how we interact with others. In fact, very little of the way our minds work is independent of social interaction. There are, of course, some psychological phenomena that are independent of social interaction—for example, the basic operation of our visual and auditory systems and simple motivations such as hunger and thirst. But anything more complex, including everything that depends on language or any other symbol system, is born out of social interaction.

Moreover, I was attracted by the idea that this intimate connection between our individual psychology and the social world begins right at the beginning of life. At that time, major new discoveries were being made in the study of very early infant development. Groundbreaking research on infants in the first few months of life was showing that infants become socially engaged well before they can do anything for themselves, and before they have much in the way of thoughts, or desires, or feelings. In the UK, the work of Colwyn Trevarthen was particularly important at that time. In the US, T. Berry Brazelton and his team were similarly influential.[7] As we will see in Chapter 3, babies interact socially with others before they can talk and before they can walk, sit up, or even control their arms. And almost from the beginning, babies are sensitive to how others are feeling. Being social is truly the first stage of being human. I knew that if I wanted to understand the nature of human psychology, I would have to study it in young children.

I published my first work on how children's understanding of concepts such as number and quantity grows out of the social contexts in which children first engage with these ideas. This line of research led me away from studying emotions such as guilt and toward a career of studying the development of social cognition. I didn't think much more about the psychology of guilt for at least ten years. And indeed, the whole field of psychology pretty much continued to ignore it. Very little research on guilt was published over the next decade.

But then one day in 1994, I was performing my weekly ritual of sitting at a table among the stacks of the university library to check up on the latest research that might be relevant to my work. In those days, before the internet, all the latest issues of the journals would be displayed together on a separate shelf in the psychology section of the library so that one could quickly survey the latest findings. I would collect up the latest issues, scan the contents pages, and photocopy any articles that seemed interesting for later reading. I picked up the latest issue of *Psychological Bulletin*, one of the premier journals for long-form theoretical articles in psychology. The title of one of the articles jumped out at me—"Guilt: An Interpersonal Approach"—and my old fascination came right back. I immediately read it.

The Relationship Theory of Guilt

The article was written by Roy Baumeister, a very well-known social psychologist, and two co-authors, Arlene Stillwell and Todd Heatherton.[8] In the article, as the title suggests, Baumeister and his colleagues proposed that guilt is fundamentally a social emotion that occurs when an interpersonal relationship is damaged. They argued that guilt is caused by the "infliction of harm, loss, or distress on a relationship partner."[9] Guilt is not simply a product of violating the moral rules of our conscience; rather it is a natural and quite basic response to harming a relationship. I was excited to read that, in contrast to the Freudian approach that humans are naturally selfish and have to be socialized to care about others, Baumeister and colleagues started from the idea that humans are naturally social; that a primary motivation for all humans is to enter into relationships with other people. Our lives are intricately tied up with others, and we all depend on others for a fulfilling and satisfying existence. While some of our interactions with others are fleeting, many of them last for years. We are born into a network of relationships, we seek them out from an early age, and we spend the whole of our lives engaging with others. Social relationships are key to almost everything we do. It is not surprising then that we value our social relationships and spend a lot of time and mental effort devoted to keeping them healthy, and that we feel bad—guilty—when we harm them.

Baumeister and his colleagues also recognized that guilt is a complex emotion. When we do something to hurt another person, there are several emotional repercussions. As we saw earlier, Freud suggested that guilt originated in a combination of emotions: anxiety over loss of love and internalized anger. Baumeister and colleagues glossed over the internalized anger part—perhaps this smacked too much of Freudianism—but they did suggest that fear or, in particular, "anxiety over social exclusion"[10] is one essential emotional element. Guilt is directly connected to the fear that we have harmed someone we care about and that there is a possibility that the other person may reject us. But, of more importance for my own thinking, they pointed to an element of the emotional makeup of guilt that I had experienced but not yet thought about: empathy for the other person's distress.

Empathy is the capacity to experience emotion that someone else is feeling. Empathy is not in itself an emotion; it is a form of emotional sensitivity or perspective-taking whereby the empathizer observes someone else's emotion and catches that emotion.[11] Thus, we may feel happy if we see someone else smiling or laughing; we may feel sad if they are somehow in distress—crying or perhaps in pain; we may even feel angry if they are angry. Almost everyone experiences empathy to some degree. It happens naturally when we observe or even imagine strong emotions expressed by others, and it is amplified when it is someone we care about. Empathy is an important part of what binds us together in relationships. We assume the emotional interests of our relationship partners. So, if a relationship partner is hurt or angry, we feel that hurt and anger with them.*

In recognizing the importance of empathy for guilt, Baumeister and colleagues were drawing on ideas first proposed by Martin Hoffman, a developmental psychologist at New York University. In an article published in 1982, Hoffman had suggested that guilt arises in childhood as an offshoot of empathy.[12] Hoffman had shown that empathy has its roots very early in childhood. Indeed, empathy for others' distress is present in rudimentary form from the first days of life. Almost from birth, infants will show "contagious crying," such that if they are in earshot of another baby who is crying, then they will start crying also. Hoffman argued that when this empathy for the distress that someone else is feeling is combined with an understanding of one's own role or responsibility for causing that distress, then the result is the experience of guilt.

Empathy struck me as the final piece of the puzzle for understanding the emotional nature of guilt. Along with the fear of rejection and possible loss of a valued relationship, the involvement of empathy allowed a place both for Hoffman's distress and for Freud's "introjected" anger in guilt. If the person we have hurt is sad, then, as Hoffman and Baumeister and colleagues argued, we will feel compassion for them, but if the person we have offended is angry with us, then just as Freud suggested, we will feel angry toward ourselves also. Guilt, then, can be understood as a combination of fear, sadness and compassion for the person we have hurt, and self-directed anger.[13]

Up to this point, I have been telling a rather dry academic and theoretical story about what guilt is and how it feels. Let's explore the feeling of guilt by using a simple, everyday example of social behavior:

---

* Empathy also occurs for ourselves. When we remember distress from an earlier time in our lives or we imagine feeling distress over something that might happen in the future, we feel that distress in the here and now through empathy.

gossiping. I am purposefully using an example of social behavior that most would not take to be explicitly immoral to illustrate how guilt can arise in our everyday lives. Gossip is a widespread social behavior that may sometimes be frowned upon but is nevertheless endemic to our social lives. Indeed, its ubiquity across societies has been interpreted by some to show that it plays an important role in the coordination of relationships within society.[14] So, take a moment to imagine that you gossiped about a good friend of yours (for ease of exposition, let's assume your friend is a woman) with a new acquaintance you were trying to impress, saying she was a bit of a flirt, and now you suspect that what you said has gotten back to your friend. How do you feel about this situation?

Most likely, you will feel guilty about what you said about your friend while trying to impress the new acquaintance. But what does this guilt really *feel* like? Certainly, your guilt is a bad feeling—the kind of feeling you would rather not have. When people describe the feeling of guilt, they often refer to a type of uneasiness or anxiety in their stomach and a kind of heaviness weighing them down, sometimes referred to as the "burden of guilt."[15] These descriptions reveal that guilt is experienced as a combination of other negative emotions—in particular, as we shall see, anxiety, sadness, and anger.

One facet of your guilt arises from thinking about how your friend will feel if she finds out about your gossiping. You imagine she will be hurt. And this is where compassion comes in. Because you care for your friend, you empathize with her distress, and you also feel sad for her. This compassion contributes to the burden of guilt—the heaviness of heart that you feel and want to relieve. You may also imagine that your friend will be angry with you for gossiping about her—a reasonable reaction. Her anger at you recognizes the fact that you are responsible for the hurt. Again, through empathy, you also feel this anger, and it makes you angry at yourself. You blame yourself for acting disloyally.

The anticipated emotional reaction from your friend to what you did inevitably generates a concern about the state of your relationship with her. Perhaps she will retaliate in some way or even cut you off. Your gossiping has created a threat to the health of your relationship with your friend. And it is this threat that generates the anxiety that is wrapped up in the guilt you feel. You fear rejection by your friend, whom you care about.

So far, I have described the emotional repercussions in connection with the relationship you have with your friend. But you may also think about the wider ramifications for your social relationships. You may worry that perhaps others in your social circle will hear about your gossiping and judge you harshly. Anyone else in your friend group who learns about your gossiping will likely be angry with you for being disloyal to your friend. They may think that although they were not the focus on this occasion, perhaps you would be just as likely to gossip about them in the future. In this way, your gossiping has put at risk not just your relationship with one friend but perhaps with others in your social network. This risk adds to the anxiety you feel.

We can see that the act of gossiping has led to sadness that you have hurt your friend, anger at yourself for acting disloyally, and anxiety that you will be rejected by your friend and perhaps others you know. These emotions do not present themselves separately but in combination, and it is this combination that constitutes the experience of guilt. Guilt is a cocktail of different emotional ingredients, including anxiety, sadness or compassion for the other, and anger directed at oneself.

If guilt is a cocktail made with different emotional ingredients, are they always mixed in the same proportions? Not at all. Every situation will be a little bit different, and one or another ingredient may be more strongly represented. Furthermore, as my own experience after the accident showed me, the same action can lead to different flavors of guilt depending on the relationships affected. My guilty reaction to the victims of the accident was dominated by empathic sadness and compassion for the extreme harm we had caused. I did not have prior relationships with them, and so there was no fear of rejection or relationship loss, at least from them. However, there was naturally a fear that many others in my world would be angry at me for my behavior. So, my sadness for the victims combined with anger at myself for what I had done and the overall threat to relationships with people at the university formed the guilt. In contrast, my guilt in connection with my friends was more dominated by fear of losing those friendships with less emphasis on compassion for their situation.

And then there were my feelings in relation to my parents. In the introduction, I described these feelings as shame rather than guilt. The distinction between shame and guilt is a subtle one and sometimes these words are used interchangeably. But there is an important difference between them. Sometimes, the anguish we feel about our role in causing distress to others is broader than just remorse for the particular action we performed. After gossiping, you may reflect on other times you were disloyal to your friends and how this pattern demonstrates that you are just not a good friend in general. You feel ashamed to be always screwing up your friendships. When the focus of remorse is oneself as opposed to the particular action we carried out, then the self-blame becomes more pervasive. We feel bad about what our action demonstrates about ourselves as a person. So, shame is feeling bad about oneself ("I am a bad person"). In contrast, guilt is feeling bad about an action one has done—the focus is on the action itself and how it was bad in some way ("I did a bad thing").[16] It is probably rare for guilt or shame to be experienced completely independently of each other. It is easy and common to think that when one does something hurtful, it is, at least in part, a reflection of our character. But there is, as we shall see in the next chapter, an important difference between whether guilt or shame dominates our feelings. With guilt, it is simpler to correct the harm. However, with shame, the sadness and anger are deeper in that they pervade the self as a whole and may be associated with helplessness and depressive feelings if we believe that we cannot change who we are.

Reflecting on all these emotional repercussions of doing something that harms others, we can see that guilt is not a simple emotion. Guilt is a complex of emotions combining in variable measures, anxiety about what may happen to our relationships both with the directly harmed party and more generally with other people we care about, compassionate feelings for the other's distress, anger and remorse about our own role in causing that distress, and perhaps shame about what that role says about our qualities as a person.

It is also the case that different people tend to react differently to causing harm to others. Perhaps you know people who tend to respond to guilt by doing everything they can to appease the person who has been harmed, whereas others focus more on self-recrimination and how they are to blame for what happened. We might say that different people mix their guilt cocktails with different proportions of the emotional ingredients. Remember that for Freud, the fear of relationship damage is combined with a large portion of self-directed anger, but for Hoffman, guilt is largely fear of relationship damage mixed with an extra dose of compassion for the person who has been harmed.

So, Freud's recipe for guilt is more self-focused, whereas Hoffman's is more other-focused. I think this difference between these two recipes reflects the reality that when they experience guilt, people may focus more on their own remorse or more on compassion for the other.[17] We do not know whether the two recipes for guilt reflect stable differences among people or reactions to different relationship contexts. I am going to call these two recipes "remorseful guilt" and "compassionate guilt" respectively, and we will encounter the distinction again in the chapters that follow.[18]

Baumeister and his colleagues' guilt paper renewed my interest in the topic. It made so much sense to me. It fit well with my personal experience in the aftermath of the accident. Here was the scientific backing to convince me that the interpersonal story of guilt was the right one. My guilt had arisen through a seething combination of sadness for the victims of the accident, anger at myself for behaving so recklessly, shame for demonstrating to the world what a bad person I was, and fear for the rejection I anticipated from family, friends, and the wider world.

Yet I still felt there was something missing. Baumeister and his colleagues' paper did not talk at all about conscience. Certainly, their interpersonal theory of guilt did not deny the idea of conscience, but it didn't explain it either.* No theory of guilt could be complete without showing how conscience fit in. The experience of a guilty conscience is a reality of life, and it reflects the fact that we all have an inner guide for rules of good behavior. Nevertheless, there seemed to be a simple solution to this concern. As I had learned from reading Freud, conscience has its origins in early childhood and is itself a product of one's personal history of important relationships. The rules of conscience arise when children do things that cause a negative reaction from those with whom they have their most valued relationships—their parents. And the interpersonal approach to conscience does explain why the guilt we feel from violating our conscience is not just about moral issues, such as hurting others or stealing. Our conscience guides us in lots of ways that aren't

---

* Perhaps this was due in part to their rejection of Freud's theory of the superego as the source of guilt.

particularly moral at all. Many people feel guilt over failures of self-discipline such as breaking a diet. I feel guilt most powerfully when I waste time that I should be spending working! It is because these expectations for ourselves were originally forged within our important early relationships that we feel guilt when we fail to live up to them. So, the interpersonal theory of guilt is entirely compatible with conscience, and in Chapter 3, we will return to this issue in much more detail.

The other important part of the interpersonal theory of guilt that Baumeister and colleagues addressed was the role guilt plays in our lives. I will turn to the function of guilt and how it motivates relationship repair in the next chapter. But before we go there, I want to consider some possible objections to the idea that guilt is founded on causing harm to valued interpersonal relationships. Let's review some situations in which guilt arises but that, at first blush, don't seem to involve causing harm to a relationship at all. We will see that they can all be brought back to caring about our relationships.

Perhaps you can recall instances where you felt guilt in relation to someone else even though you did nothing directly to harm the other person or your relationship with them. Maybe you got a pay raise and your friend who worked in the office next door didn't. Or perhaps in a company downsizing effort, they got fired while you kept your job. You may feel guilty about this situation even though you did nothing to cause it. Certainly, it is true that guilt can arise in situations where you did nothing to damage the relationship. But these situations are still ones in which your relationship may be under threat. If you get a pay raise and your friend doesn't, empathy may lead you to feel bad for your friend, worry about unfairness or inequity between you, and perhaps imagine or perceive envy on the part of your friend toward you. These kinds of circumstances can threaten the health of the relationship, even though you didn't do anything to bring it about. Under these circumstances, the guilt you feel alerts you to the possibility that your relationship with your friend may be challenged, and you might want to try to find a way to restore its health. An extreme form of this guilt over inequity is seen in the phenomenon of "survivor guilt." Survivor guilt occurs when one member of a relationship survives while one or more others perish. Survivors of war, disasters, both natural and manmade, and epidemics (such as the AIDS crisis in the gay community) commonly report guilt at surviving when many of their family or friends died. Because it is impossible to restore the health of a relationship with someone who has passed away, survivor guilt can become pathological. We will spend some time looking at how survivor guilt can lead to excessive distress in Chapter 8.

A second challenge to the interpersonal relationship approach to guilt comes from situations where we inflict harm on a complete stranger—someone with whom we have no relationship. Take, for example, my own guilt in relation to the victims of the accident, whom I did not know at all. If guilt is brought on by relationship damage, then why does guilt sometimes arise even when we do something harmful to someone with whom we do not have a relationship? There are different ways that relationships may still be implicated. First, it is important to recognize that harming a stranger might be the first step in having a relationship with them. Imagine you are at a restaurant you have never visited before and are paying the bill. You are short on funds and decide not to leave a tip for the waiter. You may feel a twinge of guilt, but it is likely that you will feel more guilty if that restaurant is in your hometown and you might visit it again than if the restaurant is in a town you are visiting on vacation and will never return to. With the hometown waiter, there is a potential relationship that has been damaged, even if at that moment there is no actual relationship. At the very least, one can imagine a future interaction with the other person in which the harmful action might have to be faced and accounted for. So, even harming a stranger may lead to a degree of guilt, especially if there is a chance you will encounter that stranger again.

Harming a stranger may also cause what we might call "collateral relationship damage." If you're out to dinner with friends and don't tip, then they may frown on how you have treated the waiter, and this may put your relationship with them in jeopardy. And then, we should also recognize that harming someone we do not know may bring in the secondary layer of guilt asserted by conscience. The rules of conscience that we acquired through our early relationships with parents and other authority figures typically include how to act in relation to others. These rules include expectations of kind or good behavior and restraints against antisocial or bad behavior. Many of those rules pertain to how we should treat others; some pertain to how we should treat ourselves. So, the guilt we feel is not necessarily in connection to the person we have harmed directly but is derived from the relationship we had with the person who first led us to adopt these rules for behavior. Perhaps the guilt we feel in connection to not tipping a waiter relates more to the standards we have acquired from our parents about not being selfish or about rewarding those who deserve it.

A third challenge to the relationship approach comes from the experience that it is quite common to feel guilt about things we do, even when it appears that no one but ourselves is harmed. This kind of guilt is familiar when we give in to a temptation that leads us away from our good intentions. Maybe we had the intention to live a healthier lifestyle, but we spent an evening bingeing on chips and pop, and are burdened by guilt the next day. I feel guilt regularly when I allow myself to become frivolously distracted from my work. I still remember feeling terribly guilty about the countless hours I spent playing video games when I was supposed to be writing my PhD thesis. I can even report that I felt guilt many times when I got sucked into doomscrolling on X and neglected my plan to work on this book! In such cases, it is the self-discipline we need to stick to a plan that has been undermined. But our own failures of self-discipline may cause no harm to a relationship partner, so why feel guilty? This kind of guilt is also based in conscience, derived from previous relationships. Self-control is itself often the internalized result of the demands originally exerted by others with whom we had strong relationships. When I think of my guilt in reaction to allowing myself to be distracted from the task of writing this book, it is clear to me that even though I am fairly "long in the tooth," it is just the latest manifestation of my conscience over being studious. It has its origins in my childhood need to please my mother, because I believed that doing well in school was the most effective way to gain her love.

Finally, how does the idea of objective guilt that comes from doing something proscribed by society or culture in its laws or religious rules fit in? How is it possible to *be* guilty even if we may not *feel* guilt? For objective guilt, the rules and norms that constrain social action are independent of any particular social relationship. For the most part, religious rules and secular laws do not specify the victim of an offense; rather, the focus is on the offense or the harm that is caused. For example, most religions and legal systems have rules prohibiting stealing. The rule itself does not need to identify whose property is stolen; it is an offense to steal from anyone. By generalizing the rule across all possible victims, any particular interpersonal relationship is removed from consideration. And without a personal relationship to be managed, the subjective feeling of guilt may no longer come into play. However, as we shall see in Chapters 8 and 9, religious and legal laws still specify how relationships between people are to be managed. Relationships between people, then, remain at the heart of religious and legal systems.

So, to my mind, the interpersonal theory of guilt provides the best comprehensive story of guilt. It recognizes three layers of guilt. First, there is guilt that is felt in relation to the experience of a threat to a valued interpersonal relationship. Guilt arises when something bad happens to a valued relationship partner that then threatens the relationship, normally because of something that we have done. Second, there is the guilt of our conscience that is felt in relation to behaving in a way that would, in our past, have been frowned upon by important authority figures, most notably our parents, with whom we had significant relationships. And third, there is the guilt that is not so much *felt* as *known*, according to the abstract societal rules against causing harm to *anyone*.

So far, we have talked about the circumstances in which we feel guilt and what guilt feels like, but, apart from a brief reference to Freud's theory that guilt guides people to act in ways that are socially acceptable, we haven't really talked about what guilt is *for*. For me, a significant clue as to guilt's purpose lay in how my guilt had been dissipated by the forgiveness of those who had been harmed through the accident. But at the time, I did not realize what this clue meant. I was simply relieved that my suffering had been lessened. To understand how forgiveness illuminated the purpose of guilt, I had to go back to school.

Chapter Two

What Is Guilt For?

In the years following the accident, I read and reflected deeply in the hope of understanding my experience of guilt—where it had come from and how it had been resolved through forgiveness—but I was not too concerned at first with why I should feel guilt or what, if anything, was the point of that guilt. At the time, it was obvious—I felt guilt because of the wrong I had committed and the harm I had caused. I was assuming that guilt was the natural reaction to causing harm, just as fear is the natural reaction to coming across a snake on a walk or disgust is the natural reaction to opening a long-forgotten tub of leftovers in the fridge. As I would frame it now, I was not particularly concerned with the "function" of that experience. It took an introduction to thinking of psychology in terms of function for me to start to ask the question: What is guilt for?

That introduction came quite soon in my graduate program in the early 1980s, when I attended a seminar course led by the well-known ethologist Robert Hinde, who was the director of the Cambridge University sub-department of animal behavior at Madingley, just outside the city of Cambridge. Hinde was tall with a shock of white hair, and he had a deep, commanding voice that conveyed all the gravitas earned from a long and hugely successful academic career. He had started out doing groundbreaking work on bird behavior. In one famous study, he described the way blue tits learned to open the caps of milk bottles, left at the doors of British houses, to steal the cream.[1] Later, he shifted his focus to primates, initially rhesus monkeys, and later great apes in Africa, where he was involved in training both Jane Goodall, who studied chimpanzee behavior and social organization at the Gombe reserve in Tanzania, and Dian Fossey, who made similar studies of mountain gorillas in Rwanda. When I met him, his research focus had shifted again to studying children's social relationships,[2] in part because he had developed a close collaboration and friendship with John Bowlby, a psychoanalyst and developmental psychologist who had pioneered research on the development of mother-infant attachment. We will meet Bowlby again in the next chapter.

It was Hinde's ethological approach to human relationships that introduced me to the importance of thinking about function. Ethology is the study of natural animal behavior, and it sits at the intersection of zoology and psychology. As an academic discipline, psychology tends to describe and explain *how* animal and human behavior, and mental processes, like thought and emotion, that underlie behavior, happen. Ethology has more of a focus on *why* animals behave in the way they do. In studying a particular pattern of behavior, ethologists will always ask, what is this behavior for? And the answer will always be in terms of adaptation—the function the behavior serves in relation to the environment that the animal inhabits. This approach, of course, is a direct descendant of the Darwinian revolution in biology—the theory of evolution by natural selection—whereby all biological characteristics may be thought of in terms of how they evolved as adaptations to the environment. Ethology is simply the branch of biology that deals with animal behavior rather than anatomical or physiological structure.

Hinde's key message in the seminar was that the environment of highly social species like humans, as well as nonhuman primates such as chimpanzees, had to be understood primarily in terms of other members of the species with whom the individual interacts. Of course, all animals interact with other members of their species for at least one function, but some, humans being the most extreme example, spend almost all their lives involved in complicated interactions with others of their species. Just think for a moment about how much of your daily activity involves others. We are in constant interaction with others. Even the apparently solitary activity of sitting at a computer and writing a book is social in that I am using language to communicate ideas with an imagined audience of readers. The reality of life lived in a social environment means that we must have sophisticated psychological adaptations that allow us to interact successfully with others. In short, human psychological characteristics must be seen as adaptations to social life.

This message was conveyed most interestingly by another regular contributor to the seminar, Nicholas Humphrey, a colleague of Hinde's at Madingley. Like Hinde, Humphrey had worked with monkeys and spent time at Dian Fossey's mountain gorilla field site. From his studies of nonhuman primates, Humphrey had become convinced that the reason primates are so intelligent compared to most other species is that their social organization is particularly complex. He had published an influential paper a few years earlier arguing that the main driver of the evolution of intelligence in primates was the need to adapt to the complexities of social life, not the need to adapt to the physical environment.[3] The requirement to keep track of the state of the various social relationships within a social group and to gain the upper hand in those relationships by outthinking one's group-mates put pressure on the evolution of ever more intelligent animals. This evolutionary pressure has been called the "mental arms race."[4] Humphrey argued that this form of evolution had reached its most extreme form in humans. He claimed that the vastly superior intelligence of humans compared to all other species had evolved hand in hand with the complexity of human society.

Humphrey's ideas were important backing for the idea that human psychology is fundamentally social. Here was compelling support for the view that humans do not have to be trained or socialized into being socially oriented; rather, social engagement is core to the nature of human intelligence. But Humphrey's emphasis tended to be on competitive interactions among social group-mates—imagine social interaction as an ongoing chess match where one is continually trying to outthink one's competitor. In such an arrangement, winning out against other people would be beneficial. There didn't seem to be much, if any, role for an emotion like guilt that was more to do with caring for others and repairing damaged relationships.

There was, however, a different theoretical approach to the fundamentally social nature of human psychology at the time. This approach focused more on positive interactions—collaboration and caring for others. According to this view, human social life is based on what is called "reciprocal altruism."[5] Reciprocal altruism is the idea that individuals engage in mutually caring, cooperative relationships with others because there are greater benefits to be gained from cooperation than from always acting alone. With reciprocal altruism, mutually beneficial relationships can be maintained so long as both partners act in good faith. But if one partner cheats, or fails to act cooperatively, then it may be in the best interests of the other partner to sever ties rather than be taken advantage of. In his foundational paper on this topic, the biologist Robert Trivers put it this way and, although this emotion was not his focus, he pointed to a role for guilt in relationship management:

> If an organism has cheated on a reciprocal relationship and this fact has been found out, or has a good chance of being found out, by the partner and if the partner responds by cutting off all future acts of aid, then the cheater will have paid dearly for his misdeed. It will be to the cheater's advantage to avoid this, and, providing that the cheater makes up for his misdeed and does not cheat in the future, it will be to his partner's benefit to avoid this, since in cutting off future acts of aid he sacrifices the benefits of future reciprocal help. The cheater should be selected to make up for his misdeed and to show convincing evidence that he does not plan to continue his cheating sometime in the future. In short, he should be selected to make a reparative gesture. *It seems plausible, furthermore, that the emotion of guilt has been selected for in humans partly in order to motivate the cheater to compensate his misdeed and to behave reciprocally in the future, and thus to prevent the rupture of reciprocal relationships.*[6]

Here, Trivers speculates that the function of guilt is to help manage and maintain relationships. It is instructive to apply Trivers's thinking to the case of gossiping that we explored in the previous chapter. Gossiping could be considered a form of cheating on an established friendship, so the guilt that arises serves the purpose Trivers identified— to motivate the gossiper to compensate for the misdeed. Now, Trivers was intentionally writing in a general way about relationships that could be applied to any animal species that live in social groups where collaboration and reciprocity are important. Humans may have the richest and most complex social organization of all animals, but collaboration and reciprocity are by no means unique to humans in the animal world. So, before we look in more detail at how guilt works to help us manage our human relationships, let's take a bit of a detour into relationships, conflict resolution, and the possibility of guilt in the animal world.

What Is Guilt For?

Conflict and Reconciliation in Animals

At about the same time that I was attending Robert Hinde's seminar, primatologist Frans de Waal published his groundbreaking book, *Chimpanzee Politics*,[7] in which he described the social organization and the power struggles within the chimpanzee colony at Arnhem Zoo in the Netherlands. This book demonstrated unequivocally that chimpanzees lived in highly complex networks of social relationships and that they were able to navigate these networks with remarkable skill and flexibility. In one episode, the aging alpha male, Yeroen, was being challenged for dominance by the beta male, Luit. One night, when none of the other animals were around, Luit viciously attacked Yeroen, causing severe wounds. The next morning, the colony matriarch, Mama encountered the injured Yeroen. De Waal describes the scene:

> When Mama discovered Yeroen's wounds she began to hoot and look around in every direction. At this, Yeroen broke down, screaming and yelping, whereupon all the other apes came over to see what was the matter. While the apes were crowded around him, the "culprit," Luit, also began to scream. He ran nervously from one female to the next, embraced them and presented his behind to them. He then spent a large part of the day tending to Yeroen's wounds.[8]

Luit's behavior on this occasion certainly looked like he was feeling guilt, including empathy for Yeroen and remorse for his own behavior. However, despite his apparent solicitousness in the immediate aftermath of the fight, Luit did not give up on his efforts to gain the leadership of the colony. He continued to challenge Yeroen, and within months, he had forced Yeroen to concede and had taken over the alpha male role.

Why would Luit show such apparently guilty behavior after besting Yeroen in a fight, particularly when he still had designs on taking the top spot in the troop? In some sense, Luit knew that there was still work to be done to achieve his ambition and, until that work was complete, he needed to keep good relations with not only Yeroen but also other members of the troop who were loyal to Yeroen. Luit was playing chimpanzee politics in the best traditions of Machiavelli.

This combination of conflict and reconciliation is a common feature of animals that live in groups. In fact, reconciliation after conflict has been reported for animals as different as sheep, hyenas, dolphins, dogs, and, of course, chimpanzees.[9] In many of these cases, reconciliation is fairly simple, involving friendly or submissive behavior. For example, in a study of domestic dogs housed at a pet food production company in Belgium, it was found that the dogs were more likely to approach another dog and lick, sniff, or try to play with that dog if they had just had an aggressive interaction than at other times. These dogs appeared to attempt to reconcile after a fight by reestablishing friendly relations.[10] But in our closest animal relatives, the great apes, active attempts at reconciliation, involving solicitous acts of caring, like Luit's, to repair the harm caused to the other are commonplace. Apes show reconciliation that resembles closely our own tendency to repair the harm that we may have done to others through our actions. So, it's not just a matter of being friendly; it's about intentionally restoring balance to the relationships in the group, at least temporarily.

Many animals in nature live in social groups. There are plenty of good reasons for opting for social rather than solitary living. Relatively simple forms of group living—such as what is seen in schooling fish or herd animals like sheep or cows—serve primarily as a form of protection from predators. It is easier to avoid being eaten if you are in the middle of a group when a predator attacks. Primates, including apes and humans, have rather more complex social organizations, living together in groups with clear roles and hierarchies. These more complex social structures yield a much broader range of benefits, including cooperation and social learning. Jane Goodall first reported that chimpanzees will work together to hunt monkeys, a particularly nutritious food source.[11] Young chimpanzees acquire knowledge of specialized tool use, such as using a rock to crack hard-shelled nuts or preparing strands of grass to fish termites out of their nests, from observing others in the troop who are skilled in the use of these technologies.[12]

Although group living confers substantial benefits on the members of the group, it also comes with risks. Living in a group means you are also more likely to come into conflict with other group members. Competition and conflict typically occur between members of the group for limited resources, such as food or mates, and this conflict can be damaging and, in extreme circumstances, even life-threatening. The most obvious and violent conflicts are often seen between males around access to mates. When such fights occur, both participants may run the risk of severe harm, which, of course, can mean that neither participant in the conflict benefits in the long run. One way that group-living animals, including chimpanzees and canines, limit the risks of such harmful conflicts is through a hierarchical organizational structure, with a dominant individual overseeing a collection of subordinate individuals, some of whom will be members of extended families but others of whom may be unrelated. Within a hierarchy, conflict is minimized because it is recognized that the dominant individual gets first access to resources, and lower-ranking individuals must take their turn. At the same time, lower-ranking individuals benefit from the protection and stability that a stable hierarchy brings. Although a hierarchical structure means that the distribution of resources, such as food and mates, is not equitable, the benefits of minimizing conflict and injury across all members of the group are worth it.[13]

Hierarchical social structures are largely stable, but that doesn't mean that there is no conflict within them between individual animals. Groups are composed of various relationships between individuals, and conflict can always emerge in these relationships. Dominant individuals regularly must exert their power, particularly when there is a challenge to their dominance from a lower-ranking individual. Individuals of similar rank may squabble as they try to eke out a living within the hierarchy. Even within closely related kin groups, life is not always harmonious. Siblings vie with each other for resources provided by their parents, and even parent-offspring conflict is common, as offspring continually demand more than their parents can reasonably provide.

When conflicts occur, reconciliation often follows. In chimpanzee troops, it is quite common for a pair of apes to get into a fight over some minor matter. For example, one animal may steal a piece of food from another, or a juvenile may vehemently resist his mother's attempts at weaning. And sometimes, there are big fights that threaten to disrupt the existing hierarchy. Luit's challenge to Yeroen's dominance was one such case. When researchers compare the amount of friendly behavior, such as grooming, kissing, and hugging, between pairs of chimpanzees, they find that these behaviors are more common in the period immediately after a fight than during other periods. Individuals are also more likely to show these behaviors to others with whom they fought than to others who were not involved in the fight. These findings strongly suggest that reconciliations are designed to reestablish good relations between the combatants.[14]

It appears that reconciliation does not occur the same way for all relationship conflicts. Frans de Waal and his associate Filippo Aureli showed that the more friendly two animals were prior to the conflict, the greater the attempt at reconciliation after the conflict. They called this the "Valuable Relationships Hypothesis"[15] and suggested that gestures of reconciliation serve primarily to protect and restore the health of the relationships that are most important to the individual. This idea means that the more important the relationship was prior to the conflict, the stronger will be the attempts to reconcile after the conflict. In chimpanzees, there is supportive evidence for this idea. For example, it is known that male chimpanzees are most likely to form strong alliances with unrelated males, whereas females tend to interact with other females in kin-based groups that are intrinsically more stable. Correspondingly, compared to females, when males fight with each other, they are more likely to later attempt reconciliation. It is possible to measure how strong the baseline relationships are between various pairs of individuals by measuring the amount of time they spend in mutual grooming and other friendly interaction. When pairs who have stronger baseline relationships fight, they show more intense reconciliation after the conflict than pairs who have weaker baseline relationships.[16] However, because chimpanzee societies are quite close-knit with webs of relationships, conflicts between two individuals often also have repercussions for others in the group. As the alpha male, Yeroen had strong relationships with many of the other chimpanzees in the group. Luit was aware that there was a danger that these allies might react badly to his challenge of Yeroen. He had to make sure that he kept on the good side of Yeroen's allies until he was sure that he could win, so he also reached out in reconciliation to these other group members.

Do chimpanzees feel guilt after conflict? We cannot really know the answer to this question. Just as for us humans, guilt does not have a clear facial expression in chimpanzees, and there is no way to assess their subjective experience. However, researchers believe that there is an emotional basis for reconciliation in animals. Conflict greatly heightens stress levels in the participating animals.[17] This stress results from the aggression shown by the combatant and the need to respond in kind to that aggression. It is believed that after the conflict ends, the experience of this stress leaves the animals with elevated anxiety about the possibility of future conflict. Anxiety is reduced by friendly contact—grooming, hugging, and kissing—which is part of reconciliation. So, what we see quite clearly is that anxiety over relationship damage plays an important role in motivating attempts at reconciliation. Just as in humans, anxiety is an important component of the experience of relationship damage and reconciliation in chimpanzees.

Before we leave our closest animal cousins, we should recognize that conflict and reconciliation can happen in various ways. For chimpanzees, conflict is noisy, aggressive, and sometimes deeply dangerous; reconciliation involves tender grooming and care. But in another great ape species, conflict and reconciliation look quite different. Bonobos are closely related to chimpanzees; indeed, they were first called pygmy chimpanzees in recognition of their overall similarity but generally smaller size and slighter, less muscular frame. However, when conflict occurs, they take a different approach to restoring their relationships. More than any other ape, bonobos use sex to reduce the anxiety created by conflict. Frans de Waal described how when food was about to be introduced into the bonobo enclosure at the San Diego Zoo, the male bonobos would get erections, and both males and females would invite each other to participate in mutual genital rubbing.[18] Similar behavior was observed in the wild when a group of bonobos encountered a fig tree laden with ripe fruit. In these cases, it appears that casual sex serves to reduce the prospects of conflict. Sex is also used as the primary reconciliation strategy. Although bonobos are rather less aggressive overall than chimpanzees, conflicts do occur. De Waal reports, "A jealous male might chase another away from a female, after which the two males reunite and engage in scrotal rubbing. Or after a female hits a juvenile, the latter's mother may lunge at the aggressor, an action that is immediately followed by genital rubbing between the two adults."[19] Of course, make-up sex is not unknown as a form of reconciliation in human intimate relationships, but bonobos appear to have taken this strategy to another level.

Guilt in Dogs?

Chimpanzees may be our closest living relatives from a genetic point of view, but they are certainly not our closest animal companions. Domestic dogs evolved from wolves, and during their approximately thirty thousand–year journey as human companions, they have adapted to be exquisitely sensitive and responsive to various human expressions.[20] We know from studies of wolves that conflict resolution occurs between these animals. Wolves live naturally in relatively stable linear hierarchies—packs—which means that there is a ranking of dominance among the group members.[21] As with other group-living animals, the hierarchy reduces conflicts among group members but does not eliminate conflict completely. Studies of wolf packs have shown that affiliative behaviors, including sniffs, licks, and body contacts occur more commonly between pairs of wolves immediately after an aggressive conflict than at other times.[22] These acts reestablish friendly relations between the previous antagonists.

Domesticated dogs that live with human owners have become part of an artificial cross-species pack, where the rules of the hierarchy are set by the human who assumes the dominant role. Under these conditions, dogs become highly sensitive to the signals that their owners send. If you are a dog owner, you may be confident that your dog feels guilty when caught in a misdemeanor. Most owners believe that their dogs show guilty expressions after being caught doing something wrong, and many believe that their dog's guilty expression makes them scold the dog less.[23] Even the founding father of the modern science of animal behavior, Konrad Lorenz, who won the Nobel Prize in 1973, believed that the guilty look of dogs reflects their guilty conscience![24] The behavioral signs taken to reflect dog guilt include a crouching or cowering posture with a bowing of the head. The dog may avert their eyes or look up submissively.*

But do dogs really show these expressions because they disobeyed an owner-imposed rule? More precise tests suggest that guilt-like expressions are no more common after a disobedient act than when the dog

---

* Readers who are not dog owners can see many examples of pictures and videos of apparent dog guilt simply by googling *dog guilt*.

is not disobedient. In one experiment conducted at Eötvös Loránd University in Hungary,[25] dogs were given instructions by their owners not to eat a piece of hot dog placed on a table. The owners then exited the room, leaving the dogs alone with the food for three minutes. During this period, some of the dogs were allowed to eat the hot dog, while for others, the food was removed so they could not eat it. The evidence of whether the dogs had eaten the food was screened from the owner's view. When the owners returned to the room, they were asked to judge, without knowing the truth, whether their dogs had eaten the hot dog. The researchers also coded the dogs' behavior at reunion. In fact, owners were not reliably able to guess whether or not their dogs had eaten the food. Contrary to their beliefs, the dogs' reunion behavior did not differ obviously when they had eaten the prohibited hot dog compared to when they had not.

If dogs' apparent guilty expressions do not reflect actual transgressions, then what are they for? Alexandra Horowitz of Barnard College in New York designed a study in which she tested dogs and their owners in four different conditions.[26] Dogs were placed in a situation where a forbidden treat was present, and their owners then left the room. For half of the dogs, she surreptitiously gave the dogs the treat to eat (which they all, of course, did), while for the other half, the treat was removed so the dog could not disobey. This manipulation meant the dogs had either been "disobedient" or "obedient" respectively. Then for half the dogs in each condition, the owners were told on reentering the room that their dogs had either been disobedient, in which case the owner should scold the dog, or obedient, in which case the owner should greet the dog warmly. Apparently guilty behaviors of the dogs, such as averting the eyes and cowering, were examined. The results were clear: the dogs showed these behaviors much more often when the owners believed that the dogs had eaten the treat and therefore disobeyed, and this happened whether or not the dogs had eaten the treat. It seems that our dogs' apparent expressions of guilt are much more likely to be anxious responses to signals of disapproval from us than an awareness that they have done something wrong. The seemingly guilty response—the cowering and submissive gestures—are there to appease the more dominant member of the pack. So, even in our canine companions, the behavioral signs of guilt occur in response to their appraisal of how well the relationship with us is going, not to what they might have done to cause conflict with us. Indeed, they may be oblivious to what they did but can just sense that we are angry with them. The guilty response may help in reducing scolding or punishment, but it doesn't mean that the same "naughty" behavior won't occur just as easily in the future.

The social lives of group-living animals inevitably consist of cycles of affiliation and conflict between individuals. Reconciliation is a critical part of these cycles. Without it, relationships would break apart and group cohesion could not be maintained. These patterns exist also in the human context. Human societies are enormously complex, but they rest on networks of relationships between individuals. These relationships must have resilience despite the inevitable conflicts that will occur from time to time.

Guilt and Apology

Different social animals have different approaches to reconciling disrupted relationships. The anxiety created from damaging an important relationship leads chimpanzees to groom, bonobos to engage in sex, and dogs to show submissiveness. These reconciliatory actions are species-specific strategies to repair and return valuable relationships to their former state. So, what about humans—how do we repair our important relationships?

The single most important mechanism that we use to earn reconciliation with someone we have harmed is apology. In his classic book *On Apology*, Aaron Lazare points to two main reasons why people apologize: "The first reason is their response to shame, guilt, and empathic regard for those they have offended. The second reason is their attempt to restore the relationship and to avoid further damage to the relationship, abandonment, retaliation, or other punishments."[27] To my mind, these two "reasons" essentially amount to the same thing—the attempt to restore the relationship *is* the response to the emotions that come from harming the relationship.

The goal of apology is forgiveness from the person that has been harmed.* Lazare goes on to articulate the components of an effective

---

* We should recognize that forgiveness is bestowed by the person who has been offended; it is not up to the offender to demand or expect forgiveness. Whether

apology—one that has the greatest chance of achieving forgiveness from the offended party. The first component is the acknowledgment of the offense and taking responsibility for it. It is important for the offender to own up to their role in causing offense and to recognize that they did cause harm to the other. It is not good enough to offer a vague or conditional "I'm sorry that you're upset," "I'm sorry for whatever I may have done," or "I'm sorry if I hurt you." A second component is to explain why one acted as one did. The explanation is linked to taking responsibility but goes further in recognizing that the person who was offended against may need to understand why the offense was caused. The third component is to express remorse with a commitment not to repeat the harmful behavior. Finally, the fourth component is to offer some form of reparation in the apology. Lazare argues that apologies that incorporate these four components provide the greatest likelihood of eliciting forgiveness. And indeed, psychological research has confirmed that effective apologies are one of the best ways of achieving forgiveness.[28]

Guilt is beautifully designed for this kind of effective apology because of the cocktail of emotions it includes. Think back to the imagined case of gossiping that I offered in the last chapter. As we saw, the guilt you would probably feel after gossiping is a combination of anxiety over possible relationship damage, empathic sadness, or compassion, for your friend's suffering, and remorse (including a dose of self-directed anger) for your role as the perpetrator of your friend's suffering. Each of these three emotional components is involved in the construction of an effective apology.

Anxiety is the component of guilt that is shared across all of the animal examples we have considered, and it is the main spur for you to act on your guilt. Anxiety is a form of fear but is more a reaction

---

and when to forgive is the prerogative of the harmed. And in everyday life, more often than not, forgiveness has to be earned. However, as we saw in my own experience recounted in the introduction, sometimes forgiveness may be spontaneously offered. Those who have been harmed may choose to bestow forgiveness spontaneously because they too value the relationship, because they recognize that we all make mistakes, or even because it is believed to be a responsibility of a virtuous life. As we shall see later, the willingness to forgive spontaneously is encouraged in many religions, and so it was with the Christian victims of my reckless action.

to an imagined threat than a present threat. We usually say we are anxious when we fear that something might happen. Fear is sometimes termed the "fight or flight" emotion, in the sense that we respond to fear either by challenging the fearful stimulus or by fleeing from it.[29] This contrast applies to the way the anxiety inherent in guilt guides us in the management of our relationships. If you value the relationship that you have harmed, then the anxiety that you feel about the threat to your relationship will motivate you to fight to salvage and heal the relationship. But, as we will also see a bit later, sometimes our anxiety over the way we have harmed a relationship may lead to more of a flight response, whereby we retreat from the relationship.

We have seen that in addition to anxiety, guilt involves compassion for your friend's distress, and self-directed anger or self-blame for what you did, what I have called "remorse." Compassion is the element that involves understanding and caring about your friend's suffering. When your friend is suffering, you want to acknowledge it and try to provide comfort. How you alleviate that distress, of course, must recognize your role in causing that distress. Certainly, it would not be good enough to simply send your friend a bottle of wine to cheer them up and then expect forgiveness.

Your remorse for being the cause of your friend's distress is what enables you to accept reprobation and punishment for what you did. Your friend and perhaps others whom you care about may judge you harshly, but you also recognize and accept that you were disloyal and that you deserve their blame. You might also accept that you deserve to suffer in some way as a form of atonement. Admitting your responsibility in this way is critical to an honest reconciliation of your relationship.

Together, compassion and remorse lead to regret—you wish you had never tried to impress your new acquaintance by gossiping about your friend. Clearly, you cannot go back in time and undo what you did, but you can express sorrow for what you did and resolve not to do it again. This regret also needs to be conveyed to your friend so they can have confidence in your future loyalty.

So, in summary, the emotional components of guilt can guide us through apology toward relationship repair and forgiveness. Anxiety over relationship loss provides the general motivation to try to restore the relationship. Compassion for the other leads us to want to alleviate the other's distress and provide some form of restitution for them.

Finally, remorse leads us to accept blame and punishment, where necessary, for what we have done and to commit to not doing it again. Together, these emotional elements can stimulate an apology that recognizes the harm caused to the other, our own responsibility in causing that harm, and a commitment not to repeat that harm.

The expression of these aspects of guilt through apology can achieve two important outcomes. First, a relationship that has become destabilized by one person harming the other becomes balanced again. Through reconciliation, the person who perpetrated the harm suffers in their turn and provides restitution to the person who was harmed. Second, there is a commitment that such harm will not reoccur. With a rebalancing of the relationship and a commitment to the future health of the relationship, the damage can be healed. This combination of responses is most likely to yield forgiveness from the other.

I've suggested in this chapter that human guilt and the way it leads to relationship recovery through apology is, in some sense, the same thing as conflict resolution in animals, so I should say a bit about whether this claim is justified. Recall that Frans de Waal and his colleagues proposed the Valuable Relationships Hypothesis to make sense of the patterns of conflict resolution seen in chimpanzees and other nonhuman primates. Nonhuman primates show more effort to reconcile after a fight with group-mates with whom they had stronger relationships prior to the conflict. Can we find a comparable pattern in humans? Recent evidence suggests that humans behave in quite similar ways to chimpanzees in this regard. For example, Yohsuke Ohtsubo and Ayano Yagi of Kobe University in Japan[30] asked students to recall an episode where they did something to anger someone they cared about. They then asked them to rate how important the relationship was to them, how guilty they felt, and whether they had engaged in an apology that included some form of restitution for the other. Consistent with the Valuable Relationships Hypothesis, the participants reported that the more important the relationship was to them, the guiltier they felt about making the other person angry and the more likely they were to offer a costly apology to repair the relationship.

It's worth noting that the Valuable Relationships Hypothesis also holds from the victim's perspective. For example, Jeni Burnette and her colleagues at the University of Richmond in Virginia found that victims of hurtful behavior by another person were more likely to forgive the other after they apologized if they had previously enjoyed a stronger relationship with them.[31] This effect was particularly strong if the apology included a commitment not to transgress again in the future. So, under ideal circumstances, guilt motivates genuine apology, which signals to the victim that the relationship is important. Recognizing the value of the relationship inclines the victim to accept the apology and forgive the transgressor.[32]

When Guilt Persists

Guilt has the right emotional ingredients to guide us toward an effective apology in the hope of forgiveness by the victim, but unfortunately, that doesn't mean that relief from guilt is always achieved. Guilt sometimes persists even after an honest attempt to apologize. Let's look at some different ways this can happen and then consider how best to resolve the guilt.

We have seen that guilt involves three main emotional components—anxiety over relationship damage or loss, empathy for the other's suffering, and remorse for one's role in causing that suffering. All three need to be working in harmony for effective action to alleviate guilt. But sometimes one or other component may be too dominant, and the effectiveness of the overall emotional reaction is diminished.

The main purpose of anxiety over relationship damage is to motivate us to try to repair the relationship. We saw earlier that one reaction to anxiety is to fight to repair a relationship, but sometimes one's anxiety can be so intense that it is counterproductive, and it leads to a flight from the relationship. Let's imagine that after gossiping about your friend, you feel so bad about what you did that you cannot imagine your friend could ever forgive you. Perhaps you told your new acquaintance, who had expressed strong beliefs on social justice, that your friend was a bit of a bigot. You didn't do it because you really believed it but because you wanted to appear righteous to this new person. Accusations of bigotry arouse strong feelings, and you suddenly realize that your friend may never forgive you for saying this about them. This is the kind of condition where the anxiety component of guilt can be overwhelming.

In effect, you believe that your relationship is fatally damaged by what you did, and so you don't even try to repair the damage you caused. Whether or not your appraisal of the situation is accurate, the inflated anxiety leads you not to risk an apology for fear of overt rejection or perhaps some kind of aggressive response that might further damage your relationship, and so the friendship becomes permanently damaged or lost. In this case, your guilt signaled to you that you ruined your friendship rather than merely damaged it. Unfortunately, then, in this case, the guilt has failed to lead to relationship repair. Without that resolution, you will likely remain burdened by the guilt of what you did, and whenever you think about it, you will feel a heaviness of heart.

A similar outcome can result for those who tend to experience their remorse more as shame, whereby they judge themselves, rather than just their action, as bad. Shame reflects a self-appraisal as bad or unworthy, and a corollary of this feeling is that we judge ourselves to be unfit for the relationship.[33] This appraisal then leads us to shy away from our damaged relationships rather than try to fix them. This kind of maladaptive reaction is why many psychologists believe that shame is an unhealthy emotion in contrast to guilt, which, when used effectively, leads us to embrace relationship repair.[34]

Now, let's turn to situations in which guilt does lead to an appropriate apology, but the relationship partner refuses to forgive. In some cases, this may happen because the partner is too deeply hurt to want to maintain the relationship. Maybe after gossiping that your friend was bigoted, you did manage to bring yourself to apologize sincerely, but they were so offended that they could not forgive you. Now, you are faced with a situation where, despite your sincere apology, the friendship remains damaged because of what you did, and so your guilt persists.

A refusal to forgive may occur because the damage to the friendship was too serious, but we should also recognize that a refusal to forgive can also be used as a tool of manipulation by the aggrieved. Perhaps your friend doesn't mind that much about being called a bigot to someone they don't even know, but, recognizing how bad you feel about your gossiping, is quite happy to extract the maximum amount of benefit from the situation and withhold forgiveness so that you will stay in their emotional debt. This kind of "guilt trip" is a useful tactic to get relationship partners to continue to try to compensate for the hurt they believe they have caused.

And finally, sometimes guilt persists even after we apologize and forgiveness is forthcoming from the person we hurt. Imagine you apologized after gossiping and your friend forgave you—are you necessarily going to be free of guilt? Maybe, but maybe not. There may be some lingering self-reproach. We can point to at least two reasons for guilt's recalcitrance. First, there may be some continuing anxiety about what we might think of as corollary relationship damage. Remember how Luit behaved in the wake of his attack on Yeroen? He not only showed caring behavior toward Yeroen, but he also made sure to show some solicitousness to others in the troop. Like in chimpanzee societies, human social networks are intricately interconnected. Your gossiping may have jeopardized your relationship with others in your social circle, who became aware of your disloyalty and revised their own attitude toward you. So, there may still be work to do in terms of shoring up these other relationships, not perhaps by way of apology directly, but certainly by demonstrating how you learned your lesson and intend to be a better friend going forward.

The second reason why guilt may persist even after forgiveness is that you remain disappointed with yourself for failing to maintain the standards of behavior you hold for yourself, such as loyalty to those you care about. Here, your gossiping was as much an offense against your conscience as an offense against your friend. Your friend may have forgiven you, but you may still need to come to terms with your own failure to live up to your ideals.

How does one deal with such situations in which guilt persists? We will return to this issue in more detail in the final chapter, but for now, let's recognize again that guilt is an emotional appraisal of the situation and a call to action. Guilt motivates us to attempt to repair our relationships, but it doesn't offer any guide beyond that. What this means is that we can sometimes remain under the spell of our guilt even when it becomes inappropriate or no longer useful. It is important to know how to let go of guilt when, despite one's best efforts, relationship repair is not achieved. When afflicted with guilt, it is valuable to reflect honestly on our responsibility for any relationship damage. We cannot direct how others choose to manage our relationship, but we can recognize that relationships are rarely completely smooth sailing; there will be bumps along the way. The key to resilient relationships is that both partners are willing to get over those bumps. If we accept responsibility for what we did and offer a genuine apology and appropriate restitution, then we should be satisfied that our obligation to our guilt and to the relationship has been fulfilled. Similarly, we may never attain an immaculate record of living according to our conscience—people slip up from time to time. At that point, a healthy approach is to commit to doing better in the future, forgive ourselves, and let go of our guilt.

In these last two chapters, I hope I have convinced you that guilt is not simply an emotional reaction to doing wrong, causing harm to others, or transgressing a rule. Guilt provides both the emotional signal that we have harmed a relationship and the motivation to try to heal the damage we have caused. In this way, guilt prepares us to respond to the circumstances we find ourselves in when we are responsible for causing harm to others. It's worth noting that this way of thinking about guilt is consistent with the modern psychological approach to emotions in general.[35] All emotions are both appraisals of the situation we find ourselves in and preparation for appropriate actions in response to that situation. It is also the conclusion that many psychologists have reached about guilt in particular.[36]

So far, I have mostly focused on the guilt that arises when we do something to hurt someone else that we care about. I have touched on the role of conscience but said relatively little about the guilt that arises through conscience. To fully understand how guilt and conscience are connected, we need to examine how both become established in childhood. That is the topic to which we turn next.

Chapter Three

The Development of Guilt and Conscience in Children

One of the reasons I have always been sympathetic to the story of guilt that Freud told in *Civilization and Its Discontents*[1] is that it resonated with one of my earliest childhood memories. Like most people, I remember almost nothing of what happened to me in the first four years of my life—the time of life in which, as Freud suggested, guilt first appears. This gap in memory, sometimes called "infantile amnesia,"[2] is because memory traces are not established during that time in a form that allows retrieval later in life. But sometime around the fifth year of life, we begin to encode events in a way that is compatible with more mature memory. We develop what is called "autobiographical memory," or memory for events in our lives that orders them into a coherent personal story.* For me, one of the earliest events in my own autobiography occurred on a bright September morning in 1963, when my mother walked me to the public bus stop with my older brother for my first day of school.

Our street was quiet, and as we passed the neat hedges and groomed front gardens of our neighbors, I strode ahead of her, excited and proud to be finally ready for school. I wore my new school uniform with knee-length wool socks almost meeting my smart gray school shorts and a light blue shirt. As we turned onto the main road where the bus stop was, we were met by the busyness of the morning rush. Cars and people were everywhere. There was a noisy crowd at the bus stop,

---

* Over many years, I have asked thousands of students in my classes to think of their earliest memory and report how old they were when the event happened. The average age is reliably four to five years. There is not complete scientific consensus for why infantile amnesia occurs, but one possibility is that before about four years of age, children are not able to think of themselves as persons who exist across time.

The Development of Guilt and Conscience in Children

including schoolchildren of all ages, thrilled to see each other again, as well as adults on their way to work. Suddenly, I felt disoriented and tiny. I clutched my mother's hand. My older brother, with two years' experience of the routine, was calm and keen to get going. He was talking and laughing with some other boys. Soon, the bus arrived, a red single-decker, number 216, and stopped in front of us. Nobody got off, so the waiting passengers started to get on. When most of the crowd was on, my brother climbed onto the bus, and then my mother ushered me to the open door and said, "On you get, dear." I froze. Somehow, until this moment, I hadn't realized that she was not coming with us. She was expecting me to follow my brother onto the bus while she went home. I gripped her hand more tightly and collapsed into tears. She urged me forward, pulling me by the arm toward the bus, but I pulled back and refused. I could not do it. All the other passengers were on board, and there was a standoff between me and the bus. The driver looked at me sadly and the door closed with a hiss.*

Suddenly, my mother was not holding my hand anymore but gripping my wrist and half dragging me home. Her grip was like steel as she marched, and I had to struggle to keep up. My arm felt like it could come loose from my shoulder. I was still in tears, but she was not looking at me. She said nothing until we were halfway home, when she finally broke her silence through gritted teeth: "I could break your little arm," she said.

Like most of the memories that people recall from early childhood, this event was emotionally intense, even traumatic, and I always suspected that it was, in some sense, formative. For Freud, this would be exactly the kind of experience that contributes to the development of the superego. I cannot say for sure that my conscience started that day, but certainly during my early childhood, whenever I felt like doing

---

* That my mother would think to put me on a public bus to go to school when I was just five years of age with only my seven-year-old brother as a chaperone might strike readers in the mid-2020s as a form of child abuse. But those were different times, predating the gradual rise in "safetyism" that dominates child-rearing in the West today. When I was growing up, it was completely normal for children to be navigating their worlds quite independently at this age. That, of course, is a different matter from whether I was *emotionally* ready for this particular adventure. Quite clearly, I was not!

something that my mother would disapprove of, I felt a pang of guilt. Most often, but not always, this internal guidance system kept me on her good side. I don't think it is insignificant that this first real threat of losing my mother's love was connected to me going to school. Since that day, the need to perform well at school has remained for me a persistent source of guilt. Maybe that is even part of the reason I became an academic!

In this chapter, I am going to look in more detail at how the feeling of guilt arises during child development and how conscience becomes established. We saw in Chapter 1 that Freud suggested a two-stage developmental pathway for guilt. But his theory had little effect on most psychologists, or perhaps it is more accurate to say that most psychologists only paid attention to Freud's story of the superego and ignored what he said about the origins of guilt in fear over loss of love. Until the 1980s, psychologists generally believed that feeling guilty and conscience were necessarily intertwined. Indeed, some still think this way, and psychologists who do not study young children regularly claim that guilt is tied to a moral sense. According to this view, the feeling of guilt depends on the internalization of moral norms and the recognition that one's action has violated one of these moral norms. The influential psychologist and educational expert David Ausubel laid the groundwork for this view in 1955, when he wrote in the prestigious journal *Psychological Review*:

> [B]efore guilt feelings can become operative, the following developmental conditions must apply: (a) the individual must accept certain standards of right and wrong or good and bad as his own, (b) he must accept the obligation of regulating his behavior to conform to whatever standards he has thus adopted, and must feel accountable for lapses therefrom, and (c) he must possess sufficient self-critical ability to recognize when a discrepancy between behavior and internalized values occurs.[3]

If guilt is essentially defined as a recognition of the transgression of moral rules, it follows that it can only arise in children once those rules are understood. This interpretation suggests that children are not genuinely capable of feeling guilt until late in the preschool period or early school-age years, when their socialization has proceeded to a point where they understand, to some extent, the moral rules of their society, and can use these rules to guide their behavior and, most importantly, inhibit themselves from doing wrong.

We now know that this is a misrepresentation of how the development of guilt occurs. Children can feel guilt from a very young age, well before they are of school age and well before they have a more general or moral sense of right and wrong. The misrepresentation comes from thinking of guilt only as a moral emotion, one that is tied to moral rules, as opposed to an emotion that is grounded in fear and empathic sadness and anger. When we allow that guilt has its basis in these simpler emotions, it becomes clear that even very young children can experience guilt.

Guilt in Early Childhood

Babies love social interaction. Other people are the most fascinating and amusing things in their world from the time they can focus their eyes. Babies will smile at people before they are two months old, and they regularly fall victim to spasms of belly laughing when interacting with people before they are even six months of age. During the middle of the first year, they take a detour into becoming interested in toys or other objects, but usually, they want to involve other people in sharing these interests, so often, the purpose of toys is to play a game with others.[4] By the end of the first year of life, babies are genuinely and thoroughly social creatures.

In the first year of life, the interactions that babies enjoy with others tend to be focused on their own interests. They are in the earliest stage of social development, which has been called "egocentric,"[5] meaning that, although they love to be with and play with other people, infants do not recognize that other people may have different thoughts, desires, and feelings from themselves. But as they develop through their second year, infants begin to recognize that others may have different feelings or interests, and they start to become able to respond to those different feelings.[6] One of the clearest examples of this occurs when toddlers observe someone else become distressed. If a twelve-month-old observes another child become upset, they may become upset themself, but they will react by seeking comfort from their mom for themself. This is more like a case of emotion contagion—catching the other's emotion.[7] An eighteen-month-old, in contrast, may observe another child who is crying, show signs of distress themself, but then try to console the other child directly, or perhaps, if their parent is nearby, recruit the adult to help. This basic empathic reaction to other people's distress shows that the emotional connection between young children and other people is well-tuned from a very early age.

Although it shows awareness of another person's distress, this empathic behavior does not reflect guilt, because it may happen even if the infant didn't bring about the other's distress. But it does provide one of the foundations upon which guilt can do its work. As I mentioned in Chapter 1, some forty years ago, New York University professor Martin Hoffman was the first modern psychologist to recognize the link between empathic reaction to others' distress and the onset of guilt in very early childhood.[8] Hoffman pointed out that if very young children are motivated by empathy to show caring for others, then situations in which they cause harm to another person will tend to lead naturally to an attempt to repair that harm. He suggested that the connection between causing harm, empathically caring about the other's distress, and the subsequent desire to alleviate the distress would constitute the earliest experience of guilt. Hoffman's idea was radical at the time, and it led to a new line of research exploring the beginnings of guilt in toddlers.

The experience of guilt is difficult to study in very young children, because they cannot yet talk about their feelings and because guilt does not have very clear facial or postural markers. Researchers usually observe young children in situations that should lead to guilt and then look for three components to suggest that the children are experiencing guilt. First, the child must be the cause of some form of harm to another person. Second, they must appear distressed or concerned that this harm has occurred—this would be the sign of empathy. And third, they must attempt some form of restitution, such as admitting the harm and attempting to repair it. These components can sometimes be observed in everyday activities, but because one can never predict when these situations may arise, psychologists prefer to try to provoke them in a more controlled setting using experimental procedures. A clever approach called the "mishap experiment" was first developed

The Development of Guilt and Conscience in Children

by Pamela Cole and her colleagues at the National Institute of Mental Health, and it has become popular because of its simple, yet effective, way of eliciting guilt-like responses in very young children.[9]

Let's look at this experimental approach and see how a typical child might respond.*

Amanda, who has just turned two and a half, and her mother, Rachel, are visiting the university child development lab. It does not look anything like the kind of "lab" the word usually suggests. It is a large but sparsely furnished room. One wall consists mostly of what appears to be a mirror. There is a small two-seater couch and two other chairs. On the floor is a brightly colored mat, on which rest a few toys. Amanda and Rachel are accompanied to the lab by a young student research assistant, carrying a bag, who has met them at the parking lot and guided them to the testing room. Amanda enters the room a little tentatively, holding Rachel's hand, and looking around vigilantly. Her mother leads her to the couch, and Amanda sits on her lap. The research assistant sits on one of the chairs and begins to talk pleasantly to the mother, who responds warmly. After a few minutes, Rachel invites Amanda to move to the mat and explore the toys, which she does. Soon, the assistant gets down on the mat beside Amanda and brings out of her bag a stuffed clown doll with floppy arms and legs. She tells Amanda that the clown is called Pat and is very special. At this point, the assistant announces that she must leave the room to make a phone call, and asks Amanda to take good care of Pat. While the assistant is gone, as soon as Amanda picks up Pat, one of his legs falls off. Now, the assistant initiates a graded series of actions to see how Amanda responds. First, from behind the door she exited, the assistant announces that she is coming back soon. Amanda looks nervous. Still holding Pat, she turns to Rachel, who is reading a magazine and hasn't noticed what happened. At this point, the assistant reenters the room, looks at Pat missing his leg, and says in a relatively neutral way, "What happened to Pat?" Amanda shows Pat to the assistant and says, "Pat broken." The assistant looks from Pat to Amanda and says in a slightly

---

* Here and at other points in this chapter, I am imagining idealized patterns of behavior. These descriptions reflect the results of these studies and are not based on actual participants.

more agitated way, "What happened to make his leg fall off?" She then looks back at Pat and, more worried again, says, "He was my favorite toy!" Still looking concerned, Amanda takes Pat and his leg and tries to push them together. She gives them both to the assistant. This whole sequence plays out over about sixty to ninety seconds. Finally, just to make sure the episode ends well, the assistant perks up and says, "Oops, I forgot. Pat was already broken. I can fix him again."

Amanda's reaction to this situation suggests a lot about her ability to feel guilt. Amanda is the immediate cause of the damage to Pat. She looks concerned when Pat breaks, and this concern increases as the assistant gets more disturbed. She knows that damage has been done and the assistant is upset, and further, she is the cause of that damage. She attempts in her limited way to repair the situation. Although we cannot know for sure, Amanda's reaction certainly suggests that she feels guilty and wants to make amends.

But can we conclude that Amanda's response reflects guilt? Perhaps she is merely showing empathy, as Martin Hoffman originally described, and trying to make the assistant feel better? To explore this idea further, University of Virginia professor Amrisha Vaish and her colleagues carried out the mishap procedure in two ways with children of two and three years of age.[10] One version of the procedure was just like the version described earlier, whereby it was the child's action that caused the mishap. In the other version, the mishap occurred because of another person's action. In both conditions, the assistant expressed the same concern about the mishap with the child. They found that the two-year-olds showed the same level of concern and attempts at reparation in both conditions. They did not appear to pay attention to whether they themselves were the cause of the mishap. However, the three-year-olds showed greater concern and more attempts at reparation in the condition in which they were the cause of the mishap. This finding supports the idea that guilt has its origins in natural empathy for another person's distress as Hoffman first suggested, and that at least as young as three years of age, children are affected by guilt, which leads them to attempt to repair the damage they have done to another person.

This early form of guilt feeling is true to the function of guilt that we discussed in Chapter 2. The guilt arises as the child recognizes that they have done something that has upset another person, and it leads the child to attempt to repair the situation. Even at this very young age, children will react to situations in which they have upset another person with an apparently guilty response that leads them toward repairing the harm they caused.

But if empathy for others who have been harmed and efforts to repair that harm reveal the origin of guilt in early child development, it is important also to note the limitation. So far, you might have gotten the impression that all that needs to happen for children to feel guilt is to show them that others have been harmed by their actions. Becoming aware of the harm to others elicits empathy, which leads naturally to a desire to repair the damage. This impression, of course, is rather an oversimplification. As any parent will report, in some situations, their children may fully intend to harm another person because this allows them to get what they want. A toddler may want the toy that another child is playing with, grab it, and reduce the other child to tears. Any concern for the other is overshadowed by the pleasure of gaining the toy. In other cases, the child may do something that doesn't directly harm someone else, but it is still deemed wrong by their parents or others in authority. Maybe the child is enjoying expressing her creativity by drawing with markers on the walls of the living room, when her parents let her know that they do not fully share her enjoyment. Or think back to the story at the beginning of this chapter. At the time, when push came to shove, I really did not want to get on that bus. It was not obvious to me in the moment that not getting on the bus would be a problem for my mother. Thinking about such situations points to a second important role for guilt. Sometimes, guilt must stop us from doing what *we* want to do when it conflicts with what *someone else* would want us to do.

The Development of Conscience

Conscience is the internal guidance system that lets us know whether we should or shouldn't do something. Although, as we have seen, a mature conscience is sometimes defined in relation to a set of moral standards, for our purposes to understand how conscience develops in early childhood, it is important to strip it down to its most basic form. When we say someone is acting according to their conscience, we mean that they understand *in advance* that acting a certain way is harmful or wrong and they are choosing not to act that way. In essence, conscience is the experience of guilt that comes from *imagining* doing something harmful to another, as opposed to the experience of guilt that occurs in *reaction* to actually doing something harmful. The importance of being able to imagine in advance the guilt associated with wrongdoing is that it can prevent us from going on to do harmful things. So, whereas feeling guilt in reaction to harming someone is important for motivating reparation, imagining feeling guilt in advance of wrongdoing leads us to do the right thing in the first place.

Psychologists have studied the early development of this role for conscience by placing children in contrived situations in which a prohibited action is tempting. One simple approach is to leave the child temporarily alone at a table with some attractive toys and tell them they cannot touch them.[11] This "forbidden toys" scenario is, of course, designed to make obeying the rule difficult. As a result, children will sometimes break the rule, and then it is possible to measure how often they do and how long it takes them to give in to temptation. These assessments give us insight into the development of conscience, and they show that conscience appears to become established at around four to five years of age.

Taylor, who is three and a half years of age, is seated at a small table that holds several toys. There is a Barbie doll, a stuffed cat, some marbles, and a shiny car. Taylor's mother sits on the other side of the room, facing away and reading a magazine. The research assistant has just left, after asking Taylor not to touch the toys because they are "special." Taylor has her hands on her lap. She looks at the toys and then looks over to her mother. She asks her mother if she can play with the cat. Her mother stays silently reading. Taylor reaches over, takes the cat, and places it on the car before driving the car over the tabletop. After a minute, the research assistant returns. Taylor withdraws from the toys. The assistant asks Taylor if she touched the toys. Taylor looks down and then at her mother. She quietly says yes. To ensure that Taylor does not continue to feel unpleasant guilt, the assistant ends the session by telling her that it is okay, and that the toys are meant to be played with.

Jasmine is four and a half years old when she comes to the lab to participate in the same study. When she is placed at the table alone and the assistant leaves, she sits very still and keeps her hands on her lap. She looks around the room and then to her mother, who is reading silently.

The Development of Guilt and Conscience in Children

Jasmine looks stiff, as if she is trying hard not to move, and keeps this position for at least thirty seconds. She glances toward the door that the assistant exited, and again looks toward her mother. She relaxes a little and quickly reaches for the cat, bringing it close to examine. At this point, having observed Jasmine's behavior on a video feed played in the adjacent room, the assistant makes a noise behind the door. Jasmine quickly places the cat back where it was on the table. The assistant reenters and asks Jasmine if she touched the toys. Jasmine looks down and doesn't say anything. Finally, again to ensure Jasmine does not carry any guilt away from the session, the assistant tells her that it is okay to touch the toys because they are meant to be played with.

Even though they are only a year apart, Taylor and Jasmine show somewhat different reactions in the forbidden toy study. Taylor shows very little inhibition. She understands that she is not supposed to touch the toys and asks her mother for permission, which she does not receive, but she nevertheless goes ahead and plays with the toys. When asked by the assistant if she touched the toys, she confesses, and perhaps at this point she feels some guilt (we cannot know for sure). However, there is little evidence of a conscience stopping her from doing the prohibited action. In contrast, Jasmine does seem to be under the control of some internal constraint. She wants to play with the toys but appears conflicted. Although she does finally give in, she is much slower to reach for the toys. For Jasmine, her attraction to the toys is pitted against the prohibition that she has kept in mind. The attraction may have won out this time, but the guidance she received from the adult certainly influenced her to resist for a while. This case illustrates the early signs of conscience as the internal force that guides appropriate behavior even in the face of a strong impulse to do otherwise.

The ability to restrain oneself from doing something that is prohibited can be thought of as the origin of conscience, but it is by no means what we think of when we talk about a mature conscience. A mature conscience is when the internal guidance system that leads us to do good deeds or refrain from doing bad deeds is more fully articulated into a system of norms or rules for "moral" behavior.

It is essentially impossible to devise experimental tasks to examine children's behavior associated with such a system of rules or norms—there would simply be too many scenarios that would need to be set up in the laboratory. So, the best way to study this aspect of conscience in young children is to use what is called a "projective test."[12] Here, children are told a series of stories that depict one person doing something wrong, and they have to imagine themselves in ("project" themselves into) the story. This method allows researchers to explore how the children think about wrongdoing and what to do about it. This approach can also probe for children's reactions to a variety of different wrongdoing scenarios, allowing a more comprehensive exploration of conscience.

An example of a story that children are told might go like this:

> Mike and Joey are playing checkers one day at school. During the game, Joey has to leave the room to go to the bathroom. While he is gone, Mike removes one of Joey's pieces from the board and hides it.

The stories cover a range of scenarios, including cheating, stealing, hurting another child, neglecting to help, and so on. Children are first asked to think about how the victim would feel, to encourage empathy for the victim. Then they are asked to take the perspective of the wrongdoer and talk about how they would feel if they had been the one to cheat or steal. Researchers review the children's responses to these questions to see whether they think the actor would feel bad about their action and whether they would try to make amends. In this scenario, seven-year-old Curtis had the following discussion with the researcher:

> Researcher: Pretend you are Joey. How would you feel when you came back and saw that one of your pieces had been taken?
>
> Curtis: Mad.
>
> Researcher: Yes, you would feel mad. It wouldn't be fair, would it? Now, pretend you are Mike. How would you feel when Joey came back and he was mad?
>
> Curtis: Bad!
>
> Researcher: Okay, you would feel bad. So, what should you do?
>
> Curtis: Put the piece back?

Results from studies of children between six and ten years old show the extent to which children at different ages reference guilty feelings (although, like Curtis, they usually don't use the word *guilty*), the harm caused to the victim, and making amends. When responses are compared across ages, we find that there are increases in both breadth and sophistication. Six-year-olds tend to have a spotty understanding of the range of transgressions and sometimes may even reference the benefits of doing the harmful action: "I would feel good because I could win the game." By ten years, however, children have a uniform understanding that all of the transgressions would make them feel bad and that they would try to make amends, perhaps by "putting the piece back and saying sorry."

These studies using projective stories show us that school-age children can imagine harming another, feeling the guilt that results from this harm, and then using this guilt to guide them away from doing the harmful act or to attempt to repair the harm caused. They seem to have internalized the rules of right and wrong and can use these rules to make judgments about what to do and what not to do. This is the core of a mature conscience.

So far, we have looked at *when* guilt and conscience emerge in childhood, but we haven't said much about what leads children to develop guilt in the first place and then how conscience takes root. We have seen that the first experience of guilt in very young children is likely based on a natural empathic reaction to others' distress. However, these empathic reactions alone cannot be enough for the development of conscience, because, although children sometimes show concern for the distress of others, sometimes they shy away from it, and at other times, children may happily do something that causes harm to another person. In the remainder of this chapter, we turn to the question of how guilt and conscience develop in children.

How Do Guilt and Conscience Develop?

An important clue to understanding how guilt and conscience develop is to look at the way children differ in their responses to situations where guilt might be involved. You might think, based on what you have read so far, that the development of guilt and conscience follows the same pattern in all children, but in fact, children do not all respond similarly when presented with these kinds of guilt-inducing situations. Even at the same age, some children are quick to help, whereas others are more reticent. Some children resist temptation quite easily, whereas others give in almost immediately. These differences among children are sometimes referred to as differences in guilt-proneness. And sometimes children show a different kind of response.[13] Remember how Amanda reacted in the mishap study by showing concern and seeking to repair the damage? The day after Amanda visited the lab, Sami, who was two and a half, visited with her mother and went through the same procedure. Sami was happy to interact with the assistant in the opening phase. However, once the assistant left and Pat, the clown doll, broke, Sami showed a quite different response from Amanda. She immediately left the broken toy where it fell and returned to the mat with the other toys. She busied herself with a toy pony, walking it backward and forward. When the assistant returned and approached her, Sami ignored her and refused to make eye contact. Sami did not appear to show guilt. And in fact, this kind of avoidance reaction is believed to show more of a shameful response to what happened. The child felt bad about herself because of what happened and so resisted interacting further with the assistant. Children who react in this way are sometimes referred to as "shame-prone," rather than "guilt-prone" as Amanda was.

Before we can say that certain children are generally guilt- or shame-prone, or that some children are more guilt- or shame-prone than others, we need to know that these tendencies occur in more than one situation and that they persist over time. For example, do children who show more guilt in the mishaps study when they are toddlers grow into children who show stronger resistance to temptation in the forbidden toys study? This question was asked by University of Iowa professor Grazyna Kochanska and her colleagues.[14] They studied the guilt reactions of children at two and then three years of age using the mishaps approach and then tested the same children when they were about five years of age using the forbidden toys task. They found that, indeed, children who showed a stronger guilt response to mishaps when they were young were more likely to resist temptation in the forbidden toys task when they were older. So, it does seem that some children really are generally and persistently guided by guilt more than others and that a tendency to experience more guilt when very young in reaction to apparent wrongdoing leads to a stronger conscience as children develop.

Why do children differ in their reaction to these guilt-inducing situations? A simple but superficial answer to this question is socialization. Children are embedded in and influenced by a social world in which other people may direct them to behave in ways that show a concern for others, and these directives ultimately become internalized as conscience. But this answer is superficial, because it doesn't tell us why children respond to and obey the directives from others. Why should children give up doing what *they* want to do just to please someone else? So, merely invoking "socialization" is much too vague to be helpful. As psychologists, we want to know *how* the social world exerts its influence on the minds of children and why the result is different for some children compared to others.

The original and most powerful agents of society when it comes to establishing children's consciences are undoubtedly their parents. Parents spend a lot of time when their children are young exerting some form of control over them. One classic study showed that about two-thirds of the interactions between parents and their two-year-old children involved the parents attempting to change their children's behavior against their will, and that such interventions occurred, on average, about every six to eight minutes![15] As children expand their social worlds outside of the home, other adults in positions of authority, such as teachers or coaches, take over part of this control. Later, as children transition into adolescence, peer groups also acquire an important role in this process of socialization. But it is parents who begin this process.

Why do children obey their parents and, later, others who act *in loco parentis*? The answer, of course, is that children love their parents, and they care deeply about protecting the love they receive from their parents. Not complying with their parents' directives risks damaging children's relationships with their parents, particularly when the parents react negatively to their disobedience. This perceived risk to the relationship elicits guilt, which, in turn, motivates children to do what their parents tell them. In this way, it is guilt in the context of the parent-child relationship that provides conscience with its power. Let's look at how this works in a bit more detail. First, we'll consider the nature of children's relationships with their parents and then move on to examine how parents attempt to change their children's behavior.

I have already described how children are social beings essentially from the beginning of infancy. Initially, babies' social behavior is indiscriminate: in the first six months, they will smile and laugh at anyone who pays them attention. But somewhere between six and nine months of age, babies start to react differently to different people. They show particular interest in those most familiar to them, normally their parents, and may cry if a stranger approaches. This differentiation among people is the first sign that babies are developing relationships with individual people. They recognize and have preferences for being with particular people. The first and most intense relationship is with the person they have spent the most time interacting with in this critical period of development between about two and nine months. For most infants, this is the biological mother, in part because breastfeeding provides a unique focus for mother-infant interaction during this period. But it doesn't have to be the biological mother. Infants for whom the primary early caregiver is an adoptive parent, or the father, or a grandparent, or even an unrelated adult such as a nanny may well develop their first strong relationship with that person. What is important for the development of this relationship is regular interaction with an adult who is attentive to the infant's needs, both physical and emotional.

This first relationship is known as "attachment," and it plays a particularly important role in social development.[16] Attachment is seen most clearly in two complementary patterns of behavior that babies show at this time: "proximity-seeking," or wanting to be close to this first attachment figure, especially when stressed, and "separation anxiety," usually seen as crying or protest when the attachment figure leaves. It is probably no coincidence that this pair of emotional reactions in connection with the parent's presence or absence usually arises around the same time as babies begin to crawl and become independently mobile. As the physical world starts to open up for the infant, the attachment relationship acts as a kind of emotional leash, allowing exploration of the space close by but from the safety of the parent's orbit.

Imagine a scene in which ten-month-old Luke accompanies his mother to a new friend's house. They sit in the living room while their mothers chat. Perhaps there are some toys strewn on the floor. Initially, Luke stays clamped on to his mother, wanting to sit on her lap or clasp her leg. But gradually, as nothing untoward seems to be happening, he becomes a bit more adventurous, perhaps tottering over to explore a toy. He sits next to the toy and examines it, occasionally glancing back at mom to make sure she is still there and available. Suddenly, the door opens, and another, older, child comes in. Luke immediately drops the toys and crawls quickly back to mom, who holds out her arms, picks him up, and soothes him with some calming words. Here, Luke has used mom as a base from which to explore the world. But if a potential threat arises, he retreats to the emotional security of this base, knowing instinctively that he will be protected. A little while later, after Luke has again become comfortable enough to be captivated by the toys on the floor, his mother gets up to use the bathroom. So as not to disturb her son, the mother quietly walks over to the door and opens it. Luke initially doesn't notice his mother leave, but as the door closes, he looks up and, finding himself alone with the other mother and child, his face crumbles into sadness and he crawls over to the door, crying. This is the other side of the coin from the secure base behavior of Luke exploring the environment. Here, Luke becomes fearfully aware of his mother leaving him and vigorously protests this separation.

The concept of attachment was first developed by the British psychoanalyst John Bowlby based on his studies of children deprived of maternal care after the Second World War. Bowlby observed that children who were deprived of maternal care became lethargic and depressed. He developed a theory about how the first relationship between mother and child becomes established and how it influences later social and emotional development.[17] Attachment is the first, strongest, and most important relationship that children develop. Human babies arrive in the world completely helpless and dependent on their caregivers—usually their mothers—for survival. Attachment is nature's way of ensuring that very young children remain safe and protected by their parents. But it is also the way children learn about social relationships and, in particular, how to relate to or connect with other people with whom they are close. For Bowlby, the mother-child relationship is uniquely important and plays a critical role in the socialization of the child. Most importantly, this relationship is characterized by the growth of love between the infant and primary caregiver. It is this loving bond, appearing before the first birthday, which provides the foundation for the lifelong relationship between child and parent. The potential loss of this love—the fear of separation—is the risk that children are most sensitive to. This bond provides both the emotional security for the child to go out and explore the world and the trust that there will always be a safe emotional haven. It also becomes a model for how children act in many subsequent relationships, including, as we will see in Chapter 5, intimate relationships in adulthood.

All children show attachment, but not all show it in the same way. After Bowlby's initial proposal about the development of attachment, his colleague Mary Ainsworth developed what became the gold standard approach for studying attachment, a procedure that became known as the "strange situation."[18] The strange situation resembles the scenario involving Luke and his mother that I described a bit earlier. Most often conducted in a laboratory, it involves placing the infant in a playroom with the mother. A selection of toys is placed on the floor, and the mother and child are given a few minutes to acquaint themselves with the room. Then, a stranger, who is part of the research team, enters the room and sits quietly in a chair for a minute before talking to the mother and then approaching the infant. While the other adult is interacting with the baby, the mother exits the room, leaving the infant alone with the other adult. After a few minutes, the mother returns to the room and the stranger leaves. There are several other episodes in the study, but this sequence of stranger approach, separation, and reunion is the core of the situation. It is designed to see how the infant reacts to new places and people, to a separation from the mother, and then to a reunion with the mother.

Ainsworth observed that most infants show a pattern of behavior in which they are open to exploring the new environment once they get comfortable. Although they are usually initially wary of the new adult and stay close to the mother, they will typically engage with the new adult after reassurance from the mother. They become concerned and upset when the mother leaves but then are easily comforted when she returns. This most common pattern is known as "secure attachment." Secure children have confidence in the strength of their relationship with their mothers, such that they do not need to dwell on it and are free to explore their environment.

A minority of infants show different reactions, termed "insecure." One group, sometimes called "anxious," "ambivalent," or "resistant," show more nervousness in the new situation and when approached by the other adult. They tend to cling to the mother more at first and are less willing to explore the room. When the mother leaves, they become very upset. However, when the mother returns, they are not easily comforted and, indeed, may angrily reject her attempts to comfort them. This pattern reflects fearfulness in the novel circumstances but a lack of trust in the mother to be the source of comfort and protection. These children are more preoccupied with their relationship with their mothers in the novel situation, which leaves them less able to explore the environment. A third group, called "avoidant," appear to be less concerned with the mother altogether. They show few signs of proximity-seeking, are less concerned by the stranger, and do not get particularly upset when the mother leaves or show enhanced interest in her when she returns. These children appear not to have a particularly strong bond with their mothers and come across as relatively independent from an early age.[19]

Although attachment style is primarily assessed by looking at how a child behaves, it is not just a reflection of the child alone. Attachment is genuinely a characteristic of the relationship between child and parent. Secure attachment is an outcome and expression of what is sometimes called a "mutually responsive orientation."[20] A mutually responsive orientation means that the parent is sensitive to the child's emotional needs and responds appropriately. For example, if the child is fussy, the parent will attempt to soothe and calm her, but if the child is happy and engaged with the world, the parent will provide suitable stimulation, perhaps a toy or a game of peek-a-boo. This kind of sensitivity allows the child to learn that the parent provides what they need—an early form of trust in the parent—and leads to a high degree of mutual warmth in the relationship. It is this mutually responsive orientation and the security of the attachment it produces that provide the scaffold for conscience to be built. Grazyna Kochanska and her colleagues have tested young children on the different guilt and conscience tasks we have looked at in this chapter and found that children who enjoy a secure attachment with strong mutually responsive orientation with their mothers show more apparent guilt in the mishaps task and a stronger capacity to resist temptation in the forbidden toys task. These studies suggest that guilt and conscience emerge more strongly within the context of a secure parent-child relationship.[21]

The child's primary attachment relationship is with the person, still most often the mother, who provides the bulk of the care and interaction with the child in the first six to twelve months of life. Of course, infants will also develop attachment relationships with others who interact with them regularly during the early phases of life. These people will include other parents, older siblings, extended family members, and daycare workers. Before long, children have become embedded in a rich network of relationships that constitutes their social group. Despite this reality, it is only a subset of these relationships—those with parents and, later, those with people who act *in loco parentis*, such as daycare workers and teachers—that are critical for the formation of conscience in childhood. These are the people who provide children with their expectations for appropriate behavior, which become internalized as conscience. So, let's turn now to examine how adults convey their expectations for how children should behave.

Parents employ different approaches or styles to try to achieve their children's compliance to their wishes for their behavior. Following a research tradition begun by Martin Hoffman over fifty years ago, three broad parenting strategies are often distinguished, sometimes called "induction," "power assertion," and "love withdrawal."[22] All these approaches communicate parental disapproval of the child's behavior, but they do it in somewhat different ways. With the inductive approach, parents attempt to guide children to behave in particular ways by explaining in a supportive manner why they should act that way. For example, parents might encourage their children to think about the impact their behavior has on others. On seeing her child snatch a toy away from another child, an inductive mother might say, "You shouldn't do that; see, you made Sophie cry." This approach directs the child's attention toward the effects of their behavior on the other child, and in the process, it recruits empathy for the victim. For situations in which the child's behavior doesn't directly harm another person, the parent might focus the child's attention on the effects of the child's behavior on the parent themselves: "You shouldn't draw on the walls because then I have to spend all day trying to clean the marks off, and that makes me sad." Here, the parent attempts to recruit the child's empathy for themselves.

The two other parenting approaches convey disapproval but without drawing the child's attention to the effects of their behavior on others. Parents who prefer to use power assertion tend to impose their will on children without explaining why and sometimes with the threat of punishment, which may or may not be physical. The child may be shouted at or physically removed from the situation. Finally, parents who rely on love withdrawal will express their disappointment for undesirable behavior or even threaten to abandon their children emotionally. In effect, they are saying, "I don't love you when you do that." My mother's comment to me after my refusal to get on the bus could be considered an example of love withdrawal, although there was an element of power assertion. In that moment, there was no attempt to help me understand my own feelings or, indeed, hers; there was just an expression of anger for what I had (not) done and a threat of physical punishment.

Researchers assess parenting styles either by direct observation of parents with their children or simply by asking parents to report on how they try to get their children to behave. What they find is that most parents will use a mixture of these parenting approaches at different times and perhaps in response to different kinds of wrongdoing by their children. Sometimes, the situation is urgent and the child must be stopped quickly. Under these circumstances, there may not be time for induction and almost all parents will use some form of power assertion. However, across all their opportunities for trying to effect compliance, different parents will often use one or another approach more commonly, exhibiting a particular parenting style.

Knowing that different parents show different styles of parenting, researchers can then examine how these different parenting styles are related to their children's expressions of guilt, either in the mishaps procedure with younger children or the conscience tasks with older children. The general finding is that parents who commonly use induction have children who look more like Amanda in the mishaps study; the children are more prone to guilt, and they tend to make more attempts at reparation. In contrast, parents who prefer to use love withdrawal are more likely to have children who respond more like Sami in the mishaps study, suggesting the children are more shame-prone than guilt-prone. Finally, children of parents who typically use power assertion tend to show neither guilt nor shame; they may be inhibited or generally disobedient when no one appears to be watching.[23]

But why do parenting strategies of the kind I have just described generate guilt at all? Why don't children simply do what they are told as a way of avoiding punishment or gaining approval? The answer is to recognize that those strategies occur in the context of the attachment relationships children have with their parents. Parental disapproval threatens the security of the attachment relationship, which most children value above anything else. So, the guilt that arises through the internalization of parental rules for conduct has its origins in the concern children feel for their relationships with their parents. Another way to put this is that guilt guides children's conduct in two ways: first, as a response to harm or potential harm to a victim, and second, as a response to harming the relationship with their parents. It is because inductive parenting layers these two forms of guilt atop each other that this form of parenting is most effective in the development of children's guilt-proneness and conscience.

We can also see from this research on parenting styles and guilt where the different recipes for guilt that we reviewed in Chapter 1 come from. Compassionate guilt that involves more empathy for the other tends to be the product of inductive parenting. Children are encouraged to nurture their relationship with their parents by empathizing with the victims of their hurtful actions. In contrast, remorseful guilt (as well as shame) tends to result from non-inductive parenting that prioritizes love withdrawal and power assertion. Here, children attempt to manage their attachment to the parent by adopting their parents' coldness or anger toward themselves when they disobey.[24]

Now, I don't want to leave you with the impression that children are simply passive recipients of their parents' efforts to control their behavior. As any parent who has more than one child will attest, even children within the same family differ in personality and in how they respond to the same parenting approaches. Research that has examined child personality in relation to parenting and its effect on guilt has shown that fearfulness, or what is sometimes called "vulnerability to anxiety," is a particularly important aspect of personality. Fearfulness can be assessed in a lab setting by observing children when they are exposed to novel and slightly unnerving events.[25] For example, the child may be presented with a remote-controlled robot that approaches them. Under these conditions, children vary in terms of how much fear they show. Some children seem relatively unperturbed by this kind of novel and uncertain event. They may approach the toy to inspect it. Other children look scared and will typically seek out their mothers for protection. Studies that have examined young children's guilt and tested their vulnerability to anxiety show that, as a rule, more fearful children seem to be more prone to guilt.[26] Although it is difficult to know for sure why this is the case, it is possible that more fearful children worry more about the repercussions of wrongdoing for their relationships, and this enhances their guilt feelings. Interestingly, when we look at how parenting interacts with children's sensitivity to anxiety, we find that the children who are the most guilt-prone of all and who develop the strongest consciences are those who are more anxious *and* who have parents who use inductive parenting approaches.[27] We will take up the link between anxious personality and guilt again in the next chapter.

I have focused here on the role that parents play in the development of children's guilt and conscience. But, of course, parents are not the only agents of socialization. As children move out into the broader social world beyond the family, they find themselves in contexts in which they develop relationships with other authority figures, who also become involved in controlling their behavior. Other carers, daycare workers, preschool and school teachers, religious leaders, coaches, and mentors all provide guidance on how children should behave. Later, in adolescence, youths turn more to relationships with peers and look for guidance on how they should behave from these relationships. Nevertheless, the same dynamic that occurs within early child-parent relationships persists. Children conform to the directives and advice of these others as they seek to manage their relationships with them.

I have explained how guilt and conscience become established within the context of relationships that children experience early in life. But I have said little about what rules come to form the core of conscience. The core of conscience is made up of the kinds of moral norms that are broadly universal and that serve to protect others from harm, things like treating others fairly and not taking advantage of them, respecting others' possessions, caring for and not hurting others (in particular, those who are close to you, such as family), being respectful and obedient (in particular, to those in authority). In many cultures, as we will see in Chapter 9, these norms are articulated in the guidance offered by religious practices, encouraged by religious leaders as well as parents who themselves follow these practices. Transgressing these moral norms leads to a potential double dose of guilt: guilt for the harm caused to others directly and then also guilt from the disobedience toward those with whom the child has strong relationships.

Guilt can also be a reaction to the transgression of norms that are more culturally dependent. These may be norms governing things such as what to eat or not eat or how much to eat, what to wear or not wear, what to study or how much to study. These norms do not in and of themselves involve protecting others from harm (although they may involve protecting oneself from harm), but they do involve conforming to the demands from those authority figures with whom the child has important relationships, and so, they can enter into conscience and become a source of guilt when transgressed.

So, we can see that the relationships that are important early in life, and particularly those with parents, act as the conduit for the moral rules and norms of society to be passed on to young children. Socialization works because children care about their parents, as well as others who act *in loco parentis*, and about keeping a healthy, positive relationship with them. Children protect these relationships by adopting the rules and norms that others set for them.

But are children simply passive inheritors of the societal norms passed on to them by others? This idea seems to clash with the belief that conscience is something personal—that we each have our own individual sense of what's right and wrong.* How could conscience be personal if it simply mirrors the values of the society in which we have grown up? The answer to this question is twofold. First, our conscience is personal because it reflects the unique set of influences that we each have experienced. When we consider the particular combination of family, teachers, religious leaders, coaches, mentors, peers, and all of the other people that in some way touch our lives, we can see that no two people have exactly the same set of societal influences. For those growing up in the same culture, there will be significant commonalities for sure, but inevitably, there will also be differences. And these differences mean that the guidance each person receives will

---

* The personal side of conscience is encapsulated by the idea of the "conscientious objector"—someone who refuses to participate in their nation's military activity for personal moral reasons.

be subtly different. So, one's conscience, in part, reflects the unique set of influences we have experienced.

Second, each of us has our own way of interpreting the influences to which we are exposed. Again, we are not passive recipients of the guidance provided by others. Different people may prioritize different relationships. One child may adore a particular teacher and hang on their every word, while their classmate may find that same teacher annoying and ignore whatever they say. And then, beginning in adolescence and continuing through emerging adulthood, people begin to focus on establishing their own individual identity. A significant part of this task is sifting through the various sources of influence they have been exposed to and determining what they feel most comfortable with. This process typically takes years and may entail embracing some parts of their upbringing, rejecting others, and searching for entirely new sources of guidance. One product of this identity formation is the development of a conscience that feels completely personal.

Thanks to the work of psychologists who have studied guilt in young children, we know so much more about the development of guilt now than we used to. We know that guilt emerges very early in life in the context of children's social relationships, and we know that the quality of the parent-child relationship, parenting strategies, and child personality are all factors in how children experience guilt and how conscience becomes established. Parents cannot completely determine how their children will experience guilt and how it will impact the way their children react to social situations in which they have caused harm to another person. But, by being consistent and sensitive to their children's emotional needs and by encouraging an inductive empathic approach when their children happen to cause harm to others, parents can guide their children to a healthy experience of guilt—one where guilt is used to heal the harm that has been caused to others—rather than an unhealthy one—where children focus on blaming themselves and perhaps feeling unworthy of love.

Children are generally highly sensitive to when they have done something to upset their parents. When parents signal their disapproval, children naturally interpret it as a threat to the quality of the relationship with their parents, and they will harbor guilt as a result. So, one of the very best parenting practices is to always leave an encounter where control and discipline must be meted out with an assurance that, nevertheless, the child is loved. In a sense, this assurance is a sign of forgiveness for what the child may have done. In this way, the child's guilt over harming their relationship with their parents is not able to fester and build with every misdeed.

But even with the best of intentions, parenting for the development of healthy guilt can be difficult. In the rough and tumble of everyday life, it's so easy for a parent to let a comment slip that might be received by their child as a threat of punishment or love withdrawal. And it's interesting to me how one comment made in a moment of frustration can have a profound effect.

When I was reviewing the research I have described in this chapter, my mind again went back to the episode at the bus stop. I was at exactly the age at which the research we have just reviewed has shown that conscience is developing. Faced with the prospect of getting on the bus without my mother, to whom I was strongly attached, I was gripped by extreme anxiety; I just could not bring myself to embark on this adventure while leaving her behind. Yet, in acting this way, I had angered my mother and thereby jeopardized my relationship with her. My mother, who was a homemaker at the time, had three children within four years of each other, including my older brother and younger sister. On this occasion, like any parent of three small children after a long summer, she was probably at her wits' end and was likely relishing the relief that would come from two of them being taken care of during the school day. Her plans for that day had been frustrated and she would now have to look after me. My mother was not a cruel woman—far from it. She was generally devoted and caring. Her parenting was firm with clear rules for conduct, but not harsh, unreasonable, or inconsistent. Like most middle-class British parents of a certain vintage, she was not overly warm and probably leaned toward assertive parenting rather than inductive. She certainly was keen to encourage independence. Of course, at the time, I knew none of this. I was only aware of the intense emotions at play. I was terrified of the impending separation from my mother at the bus stop, and I was embarrassed in front of the bus driver and the passengers looking at me. At that moment, I needed tenderness from my mother, but what I got was anger and a threat that suggested she didn't love me. So, on top of my separation anxiety and embarrassment, I got another shot of fear—if

The Development of Guilt and Conscience in Children

I didn't do what she wanted, my bond with her was under threat. I knew that I was the cause of my mother's anger for not doing what she wanted me to do. I learned something that day about disobedience, that it carried a very real threat of rejection and even violence—I felt it in the way my mother dragged me home and in the words she spoke. Most disturbingly, I learned that my relationship with her was precarious and that I had better do what she wanted if I did not want to lose her love. To protect my relationship with my mother, I had to overcome my anxiety. I believe a cornerstone of my conscience was laid that day, as my need to do what she wanted me to do became more powerful than my natural desires or fears. The next day, my mother walked me to the bus stop again. When the bus arrived, I followed my brother up the steps, and as I sat down next to him, I heard the hiss of the bus door closing behind me.

Chapter Four

Guilt-Proneness

The school bus experience I related in the last chapter left a peculiar legacy on my psyche. Even now, some sixty years later, I experience guilt about not working hard enough. I have been an academic psychologist for forty years and I have had a reasonably successful career. I have published a significant amount of original research, trained many students, and served as chair of my academic department and dean of my faculty. I have attained all the goals I set for myself when I was a graduate student—and more. Surely, by now, I should be able to work (or not work) when I want?

But no, I remain particularly prone to feeling guilt in connection to my work. If I am not working, there is an internal voice (hi, Mum!) nagging me to get back at it. I am, at least in my work life, what we call "guilt-prone."

It's clear that people differ greatly in how much they feel guilt, and some, it seems, feel no guilt at all. Just as I was preparing to write this chapter on how people feel guilt to differing degrees, a notification came through my X feed alerting me to a newly published essay in the leading medical journal *The Lancet*,[1] recognizing the eightieth anniversary of the initial publication of the first edition of Hervey Cleckley's book on psychopathy, *The Mask of Sanity*.[2] I had read Cleckley's book about thirty years earlier, when I was looking into the relevance of psychopathy for my own research on the psychology of social relationships, and it was nice to be reminded of its relevance for our field. Few scientists enjoy the level of respect and notoriety in their disciplines that their contributions are celebrated decades later.

But Cleckley's work remains significant because it essentially ushered in and defined the modern era of the scientific study of psychopathy.*

After a stellar academic training, including a Rhodes scholarship at Oxford University, Cleckley received his MD in 1929 and spent the next dozen years practicing psychiatry in hospitals around Augusta, Georgia. There, he was struck by a type of patient who appeared quite sane and yet was completely unable to lead a functional and successful life. Cleckley became convinced that beyond the traditional types of madness, such as the delusions of psychosis or the extreme anxiety of the neuroses, there was another form of mental illness, characterized not by disturbed consciousness, but by a fundamental and pathological lack of social and emotional skills lurking underneath an apparently normal consciousness—hence the title of his book.

To illustrate his theory of psychopathy, Cleckley presented several lengthy case histories of individuals he had worked with. Many of these cases came from apparently healthy and supportive families who could not understand why the individuals involved were so intent on causing such distress to them and others. He avoided describing psychopaths who had committed extreme acts of violence, such as torture of pets in childhood or murder and rape as adults, because he did not want the reader to get distracted by the excesses of such antisocial behavior. His goal was to elucidate the life history of psychopaths from a psychological point of view, not simply to condemn their egregious lifestyles.

The portraits of these cases are exquisitely drawn by Cleckley, and I recommend reading them.[3] I particularly like the case history of Tom, as it captures the essence of psychopathy so well. As with many psychopaths, Tom's abnormal behavior appeared quite early in childhood as a string of disobedient, reckless, and seemingly pointless acts. As a child, Tom stole silverware and clothes from his family and sold them for a pittance. At school, he regularly caused fights for no reason, and he

---

* Cleckley used the term "psychopathy," and this term is used most consistently in the psychological and psychiatric literature. Some authors prefer the term "sociopathy," and, in fact, I also prefer this term, because it reflects what I think is the fundamental nature of the condition, that of a profound disturbance of social relationships—a social pathology—rather than a more general psychological pathology. However, I retain the term "psychopathy" in this chapter to be consistent with the more common use.

defecated in the school piano just for a prank. Tom always denied his wrongdoing with such conviction and seeming honesty that he was often believed, until the evidence was clear that he was the culprit. At this point, he would apologize with apparent sincerity and vow never to do such things again. He was able to put on such a good show of contrition that he would charm his parents and teachers. He would then do exactly the same kinds of things the next day or week.

This pattern persisted throughout his childhood, and he never seemed to learn. Gradually, throughout adolescence, the seriousness of his delinquency increased. At one point, Tom got into trouble with the law for stealing a car. He was put on probation after his first offense, but immediately stole another car for no good reason, at which point he received his first prison sentence. He was let out early after showing good behavior and a reformed attitude and was able to find a menial job. However, at work, he arrived late and sometimes did not appear for no reason. He quit after a short time, saying that he just didn't want to work anymore. By early adulthood, it was estimated that Tom had been arrested fifty or sixty times, mostly for minor offenses. And there were many more incidents that did not result in legal trouble because his family made excuses for him.

Like many psychopaths, Tom had a highly abnormal history of romantic relationships. His sexual desire and superficial charm led him to engage with women, but he showed no inclination to care about them or develop anything resembling a mutually responsive relationship. He did marry a prostitute, for whom he also acted as a pimp, but deserted her after a brief time. He then took up with the wife of a serviceman who was on active duty, as well as (concurrently) a series of other women. With all these women, he enjoyed sexual encounters but never showed qualms about moving on to the next sexual interest. The fact that he was able to entice a series of women into sexual encounters suggests some degree of masculine charm, but like everything else in his life, his approach was entirely superficial, designed for short-term gain.

Tom illustrates three aspects of psychopaths' way of life. First, psychopaths fail to respect relationships right across the board. They disdain, neglect, and generally take advantage of parents, acquaintances, lovers, and authority figures in equal measure. Second, the abuse of these various relationships occurs repeatedly over an extended period and never seems to improve (despite common expressions of regret and commitments to change). These are not occasional or momentary lapses of caring for others, but a protracted failure to nurture relationships over weeks, months, and years. Third, long-term neglect contrasts with short-term attention to others, in an often charming and convincing manner, to placate them or manipulate them into serving their immediate needs.

When I first read the case histories in Cleckley's book, I was astonished. Sometimes, a phenomenon is best observed through its absence. If we put aside for a moment the obvious delinquent and criminal behavior so characteristic of psychopaths, what Cleckley was describing in his subjects like Tom was the complete absence of a normal human approach to social relationships. Most of us exist willingly and enthusiastically within a network of social relationships, many of which are very long-lasting. So much of what we aspire to in life—healthy relationships with our family, fulfilling social lives, and satisfying careers—depends on our ability to forge mutually beneficial relationships. We have relationships with the members of the family that we grew up in—parents, siblings, grandparents, aunts, uncles, and cousins. We have relationships with lovers and spouses and our own children. We have relationships with friends, those we work with, and those we worship alongside. We spend considerable effort ensuring that these relationships remain healthy even when they inevitably hit the occasional bump in the road.

The life history of psychopaths like Tom is what human existence looks like when the natural inclination to cultivate such a network of social relationships is missing. Take away the motivation to build a life based on relationships and this is what you get. Psychopaths are completely focused on their own immediate, often idiosyncratic interests; other people only serve as short-term means to further these interests. The antisocial behavior they show—the stealing, lying, manipulation, and general unreliability—is, at least in part, a by-product of the fact that psychopaths just don't care about other people! Sometimes, this antisocial behavior plays out in the extreme and gratuitous violence of famous psychopaths such as Ted Bundy (especially when the psychopath comes from a family with a history of violence), but sometimes, it plays out simply in the complete disinterest in, and therefore neglect of, the concerns of others.

What is missing in the psychological makeup of psychopaths to make them so oblivious to the management of their social relationships? Cleckley emphasized, among other characteristics common to his patients, certain core emotional features. In particular, he identified a general emotional unresponsiveness, including an absence of nervousness or anxiety and a lack of remorse or shame. In short, Tom and his ilk appeared to lack the essential emotional bases for caring about and maintaining social relationships—the critical components of guilt.

As I noted earlier, Cleckley's characterization of psychopathy was highly influential in the development of subsequent clinical work. The most widely used and validated assessment for psychopathy in use today, the Psychopathy Checklist Revised (PCL-R), was designed by Canadian psychologist Robert Hare, drawing broadly on Cleckley's work.[4] A key component of the PCL-R is the assessment of guilt or remorse, empathy, and self-blame—the emotional elements of the guilt "cocktail" I described in Chapter 2. Psychopaths show abnormally low levels of these emotional reactions. It is now generally believed that a fundamental core feature of psychopathy is an absence of the emotional underpinnings of successful social relations—empathy, remorse, and guilt—and an associated absence of anything like a moral compass. In his own book on psychopathy, Robert Hare refers to psychopaths as "without conscience."[5]

However, because the absence of these social emotions is difficult to measure, some in the psychiatric community prefer to rely on more objective measures such as persistent criminality, which is more easily recorded.* Robert Hare developed the PCL-R while working with prison inmates, because that population has a large proportion of psychopaths, and his measure also assesses criminal behavior. From his research, Hare suggested that there are two superordinate dimensions of psychopathy, and people can vary from low to high on both.

---

* Sometimes, psychopathy is referred to as "antisocial personality disorder" in recognition of the fact that psychopaths act in antisocial ways broadly and repeatedly. But most clinicians prefer to distinguish antisocial personality disorder from psychopathy, because some people commit repeated antisocial acts as a result of abusive conditions of upbringing that lead them to harbor broad-based anger directed at society rather than because of a profound lack of social emotions.

One dimension covers the "Interpersonal/Affective" characteristics and includes the psychopath's lack of remorse and empathy, as well as the deceptive and manipulative interpersonal behavior. The other dimension covers the "Lifestyle/Antisocial" characteristics, including the lack of long-term plans, need for stimulation, impulsivity, as well as the criminal behavior. If we reflect for a moment on the two types of definition of guilt mentioned in the introduction, we can say that these two dimensions reflect an increased tendency to be *objectively guilty* of wrongdoing in the absence of any *subjective guilt* about that wrongdoing. Not surprisingly, the absence of the experience of guilt is linked to the presence of antisocial behavior.

Clearly, most psychopaths who come to the attention of the legal system do so because of their recklessness and tendency to engage in delinquent or criminal activity. Even if they are not disposed toward violence, many psychopaths show a persistent pattern of petty criminality like Tom. The popular image of the psychopath as a violent criminal or serial killer has arisen largely because these are the most morbid and newsworthy cases. But psychopathy need not be associated with violence or criminality. In his original work, Cleckley described a number of cases of psychopaths living in the general population, undetected in the sense that they had no criminal record and were not receiving psychiatric interventions. Hare has suggested that the psychopathic disregard for others' feelings and the associated skill at social manipulation may allow psychopaths to be more successful than the average person at climbing the corporate ladder.

It may be that female psychopaths, being naturally less prone to recklessness and physical aggression, show less criminal activity and so are less likely to be identified.[6] In her memoir *Confessions of a Sociopath*,* M.E. Thomas relates how she has lived successfully as a psychopath, staying on the right side of the law, while showing the same disregard for social relationships as Cleckley described in his patients.[7] Thomas recounts how, on reading *The Mask of Sanity*, she saw herself

---

* M.E. Thomas also prefers the term "sociopath" to avoid the association of "psycho" and its connotations of violence. Thomas has no inclination to violence, despite her lack of interest in social relationships.

in Cleckley's descriptions. Her remarkable self-awareness and autobiographical skill provide a first-person perspective on psychopathy that is unparalleled and, as she herself attests, completely consistent with Cleckley's clinical third-person descriptions. She admits to having no meaningful experience of guilt or empathy, writing, "Normal people feel emotions that I simply don't. For them, emotions like guilt serve as convenient shortcuts, telling people when they're crossing societal or moral boundaries. But guilt is not absolutely necessary to live within social acceptability."[8]

If you take away the criminality (and the associated need for either psychiatric or criminal justice interventions) in the lives of psychopaths, how should we regard this condition? Perhaps it becomes reasonable to regard psychopathy as a particular way of being in the world, one that is lacking in the social emotions, including guilt, that bind people to others. Their social lives are not governed significantly by guilt in the way that other people's lives are, and without this emotion, psychopaths place less value on managing their social relationships than most people.

Viewing psychopathy this way shows us that we should consider guilt not only as a reaction to a particular instance of doing something to harm a relationship but also as a general tendency to experience this emotion in a range of situations and across the lifespan. The role of guilt in our lives is not just to help manage conflict in a relationship; it is to help cultivate the health of our *many* relationships over time. To clarify this distinction, psychologists sometimes refer to the difference between "state" and "trait" guilt. State guilt is a particular experience of guilt, such as feeling guilty about gossiping about a friend, whereas trait guilt is the tendency to feel guilt across a range of different circumstances. When a person tends to experience guilt in all kinds of different circumstances, such as with family, friends, at work, and so on, and when this tendency to feel a lot of guilt persists over time, then we refer to it as a personality trait.

In contrast to psychopaths, who feel almost no guilt, the average person has a disposition to feel some guilt regularly through their lives and in connection to a variety of relationships. But thinking about people as "average" masks a lot of variability in the tendency to feel guilt. You probably know some people who seem to feel guilt a lot of the time, in all kinds of circumstances, and even perhaps when it is not really warranted. Perhaps you are one of those people. And then there are others who are relatively free from guilt and only experience it when they have clearly done something to harm another person that they care deeply about. Sometimes, we talk about this disposition as "guilt-proneness," meaning how likely a person is to feel guilty in any particular circumstance. If guilt-proneness is a continuum of the tendency to feel guilt, psychopaths are at one extreme end—they never feel guilt—and the rest of us fall at some other point on the remainder of the continuum.

Individual Differences in Guilt-Proneness

Why are some people very guilt-prone and others not so much? You may have heard about the "nature versus nurture" distinction that is often used to try to answer this kind of question. Is being prone to guilt something we are born with or something that we are socialized into? Psychologists often point to two broad sets of influences when thinking about how people come to be the way they are. One set includes the individual experiences that people encounter as they go through life, and in particular, the experiences they have growing up through childhood. This is the *nurture* side.

The other set is the predispositions that are provided by *nature*. It is a common misconception to assume that the set of predispositions provided by nature is narrowly the product of the genetic makeup of the person. I want to emphasize that this is inaccurate. Certainly, genetic variation can and does contribute to psychological differences, but "nature" also includes the relatively fixed environment, sometimes called the "shared environment," that people in a particular group encounter. What this means is that members of one group of people may differ from the members of another group of people not because the groups are genetically different, but because the members of one group are all exposed to a set of experiences that are shared by all members of the group and are different from the set of experiences encountered by all members of the different group. Shortly, we will take a look at three aspects of nature that appear to be connected to guilt-proneness: general personality, gender, and culture.

But first, we need to explain how psychologists go about measuring people's guilt-proneness. As with most aspects of personality, psychologists rely heavily on people's responses to carefully designed questionnaires to measure guilt-proneness. These questionnaires typically require people to report on whether they would feel guilty in a variety of hypothetical scenarios. Usually, several different scenarios are presented and then an overall assessment of guilt-proneness is determined. In the simplest sort of measure, people are asked to imagine doing offensive or illegal things and then simply rate how guilty they would feel on a numerical scale, perhaps from 1, meaning not guilty at all, to 5, meaning extremely guilty. For example, one scenario might be: "How guilty would you feel if you stole something from a store worth fifty dollars, even if no one found out?"

A richer approach is to contrast a guilt reaction with other possible reactions to different scenarios. The most popular measure of this kind currently in use is called the Test of Self-Conscious Affect (TOSCA).[9] Respondents are presented with a series of short descriptions of an event, and they must judge the extent to which they might experience each of four reactions. Here's one example of the sixteen scenarios in the TOSCA:

While out with a group of friends, you make fun of a friend who's not there.

> A. You would think: "It was all in fun; it's harmless."
>
> B. You would feel small...like a rat.
>
> C. You would think that maybe that friend should have been there to defend him/herself.
>
> D. You would apologize and talk about that person's good points.

Respondents are asked to rate each of those statements from 1 (not likely) to 5 (very likely). The four statements reflect four possible attitudes to the scenario. For this example, (a) reflects a *detached* reaction, because that response does not engage with the disloyalty and the possible hurt feelings of the friend; (b) reflects *shame*, because the focus is on your qualities as a friend and as a person; (c) reflects *externalization*, because any blame is placed outside the self; and (d) reflects *guilt*, because the response is one in which you take responsibility for your potentially hurtful action and try to provide restitution.

Guilt-Proneness

After rating all possible responses to all sixteen scenarios, participants are assigned a summary score for guilt-proneness as well as for shame-proneness, detachment, and externalization. So, as you might expect, people who show psychopathic tendencies also show low levels of guilt-proneness.[10]

General Personality and Guilt-Proneness

The idea that people differ from each other in general and consistent habits of mind has been around for millennia. Hippocrates, the Greek physician of the fifth century BCE, whose oath (at least in modified form) is still repeated by medical students today, believed that there were four personality types reflecting which of four bodily fluids—blood, yellow bile, black bile, and phlegm—was most dominant in the body. These days, the so-called five-factor, or "Big Five," model of personality is the approach that has most consensus among psychologists. According to this model, general personality is best understood as a combination of five main traits. For ease of remembering, these are sometimes combined into the mnemonic *OCEAN*.[11] The five factors are outlined in the table on the next page.

These traits describe the enduring and consistent ways that people behave. This means that people tend to show similar patterns of behaviors over time and across different situations. They are somewhat, although not completely, independent dimensions of personality, which means that a person can be high or low or in-between on any of them, and where you fall on one trait has relatively little to do with where you fall on any other trait.

TRAIT	DESCRIPTION	
	HIGH	LOW
OPENNESS	Openness to new ideas and challenges; creative and imaginative	Concrete thinker; resistant to change and new ideas

CONSCIENTIOUSNESS	Organized; planful; detail-oriented; prefer structure	Spontaneous and impulsive; disorganized; flexible; resistant to structure
EXTRAVERSION	Sociable, assertive, emotionally expressive	Prefer solitary activities; find socializing tiring; dislike being the center of attention
AGREEABLENESS	Caring of others, helpful, compliant, trusting, make friends easily	Not interested in others' concerns, competitive, distrustful
NEUROTICISM (EMOTIONAL STABILITY)	Easily stressed, anxious, moody	Calm, bounces back from upset quickly, generally happy

These five personality factors have been found to be quite consistent in adults. That is, your tendency to be extraverted, conscientious, or agreeable remains about the same throughout adulthood.[12] That is not to say that people's personalities cannot change at all throughout life. But it does mean that your personality is not completely malleable. For example, if you are an introvert, while you can learn the social skills that come naturally to extraverts, you will always lean toward solitary activities and get tired from social engagement.[13]

Psychologists believe that different emotions are essential ingredients of these different personality dimensions. For example, extraversion is related to a generally happy disposition, whereas neuroticism is related to anxiety and sadness. So how does guilt-proneness connect to these general dimensions of personality? The first people to look at this question about twenty-five years ago were Danielle Einstein, who began the research as an undergraduate student in Australia, and her advisor, Kevin Lanning.[14] Einstein and Lanning used several different measures to assess guilt-proneness, including the TOSCA. From the way their participants responded, they were able to distinguish two components of guilt-proneness—empathic guilt and anxious guilt—as well as shame-proneness. These three emotional aspects of guilt correspond to the different emotional components of guilt that I introduced in Chapter 2.

Empathic guilt is the feeling of guilt that is more dominated by a reaction to the harm caused to others; it is similar to what I called "compassionate guilt." Anxious guilt is guilt that is more dominated by fear of a threat to their relationships. Shame-proneness is more of a reaction to how doing something harmful to others would make people feel about themselves. When Einstein and Lanning looked at how these different aspects of guilt relate to the Big Five personality factors, they found that people who reported empathic guilt tended to score highly on agreeableness, whereas those who reported anxious guilt and shame had higher scores on neuroticism.

Since Einstein and Lanning's study, several researchers have examined the link between guilt-proneness and personality. These subsequent studies with people from different countries around the world have strongly confirmed the link between guilt-proneness and agreeableness.[15] People who are high on agreeableness generally care about others, both in terms of looking out for their interests and in terms of relieving their distress. They are helpful and cooperative, and they believe that others are honest and trustworthy. They are willing to sacrifice their own interests to keep others happy. In short, they have a personality that orients them toward seeing others in the best light and to getting on with other people. It makes good sense, then, that they feel bad when they hurt someone else and that they will try to make things right. Guilt is one of the emotions that is well suited to the agreeable person's life!

The connection between neuroticism and guilt-proneness has also received additional support.[16] This connection also makes sense if we remember that guilt has an anxiety component—we feel guilt when we worry that we have damaged a relationship. People who tend to have higher anxiety in general are likely to worry more about their relationships, and this could make them more prone to guilt. However, chronic anxiety may also lead people to shy away from attempting to heal their relationships, and in line with this idea, research has shown that people who score very high on neuroticism show more shame-proneness than guilt-proneness.[17]

The other of the Big Five factors that has been found to be reliably linked to guilt-proneness is conscientiousness.[18] This connection should also be no surprise. After all, the word *conscientious* is derived from *conscience*, and its original meaning was related to knowing right from wrong. In its modern usage in personality theory, conscientiousness is broader than a sense of morality. Conscientious people show high levels of self-discipline and responsibility in general, not just in relation to moral issues. They play by the rules and are dependable or reliable. They set goals and work to achieve them in an organized, planful way.

Because of this approach to life, high conscientiousness is often thought to be a desirable trait in work and school contexts. Guilt is one of the emotional drivers that allows conscientious people to maintain their careful and ordered approach to their lives. Remember that conscience is derived from the rules that were once handed down to us by authority figures with whom we had important relationships, such as our parents. These rules become internalized as conscience, so that when we fail to live up to them, or even imagine not living up to them, we can be hit by the guilt originally associated with not being obedient or meeting the standards that were set for us.*

Gender Differences in Guilt-Proneness

It is something of a stereotype (at least in Western culture) to assume that women are more emotional than men—particularly when it comes to the social emotions like guilt, shame, empathy, and embarrassment. But is there actual evidence to support this stereotype? Essentially, all studies that have looked at guilt-proneness using measures like the TOSCA record the gender of the participants, even if gender differences were not the focus of the study. Because of this, there is now a very large

---

* I should point out that guilt-proneness is not related to all personality dimensions. It has not been shown to be related to either openness or extraversion in any studies. If guilt-proneness was linked to any and all personality dimensions, then personality would not be particularly helpful in understanding the nature of guilt.

database of results that allow us to examine the extent of any difference in guilt-proneness between women and men.

In 2012, psychologist Nicole Else-Quest and her colleagues published a meta-analytic review of all available published and unpublished studies on several self-conscious emotions, including guilt, shame, pride, and embarrassment, that reported gender comparisons.[19] A meta-analysis is essentially a single combined analysis of many different studies that looks for reliable patterns in the results when all the studies are considered together. After reviewing well over two hundred different studies, involving thousands of participants, they found that there are clear gender differences for both guilt- and shame-proneness, such that women are more disposed to feeling guilt and shame across different situations than men. This difference was not found for embarrassment or pride, so it is not that women experience more self-conscious emotion generally; it is more specific to guilt and shame.

Now, this does *not* mean that all women experience more guilt than all men. It is an average difference. There are plenty of women who experience less guilt than the average man. But it *does* mean that there is something about being a woman that predisposes a person to be likely to feel more guilt than a man. Interestingly, the gender difference only appears for adolescents and adults; studies on guilt-proneness show no gender differences for younger children. So, there seems to be something about the transition to adulthood that leads to a differentiation in guilt experience for males and females.

Why might women experience more guilt than men? There are likely several interconnected reasons. First, it is well-known that, on average, women score more highly than men on the personality dimensions of agreeableness, neuroticism, and conscientiousness. As we have already seen, these personality attributes are connected to a greater concern for relationship management and to more experience of guilt. Second, the concern for relationship management is encouraged through cultural expectations. Women are expected to be more focused on maintaining the health of friendship and family networks. And finally, women tend to connect with others in ways that require more focus on individual relationship management. Several research studies comparing women's and men's patterns of social relationships have found gender differences in relationship networks. In general, women tend to relate to others more in terms of one-on-one friendships, which are closer and more intimate, and typically require more emotional investment, whereas men interact more commonly in groups, which require less individual investment to achieve the health of the group dynamic. An international team of researchers led by Robin Dunbar of the University of Oxford found an ingenious way to get a massive sample of data to test this pattern across many ethnic groups and different cultures. They compared over 100,000 Facebook profile pictures drawn from many different geographic regions and looked specifically at profile pictures with more than one person in them. The idea is that profile pictures reflect the kinds of social activity the profile holder engages in. They found that for women, when the profile picture contained more people than just the profile holder, it was most common for there to be just one other, usually female, person. In contrast, when men used a profile picture with more than just themselves, it was more likely to be a group photo. This difference was seen in all the geographic regions sampled, including Africa, Asia, Australia, Europe, Latin America, and North America, so it is not a pattern that is specific to one culture. As they say in the title of their paper: "Women Favour Dyadic Relationships, but Men Prefer Clubs."[20]

Men's social lives might appear to involve larger group relations than those of women, but both men and women have close one-on-one relationships, including their romantic partnerships and their closest friends. A general finding is that women have higher levels of intimacy with their friends than men do. For example, in a very recent study using online research forums, Dunbar's research group asked a large sample of men and women, drawn mostly from Europe and North America, to reflect on their relationship with their romantic partner and their best friend, defined as "the nonrelated person who you would turn to first, after your romantic partner, during a time of extreme difficulty or emotional distress." On average, women reported much higher intimacy with both romantic partners and best friends than men. Interestingly, and perhaps surprisingly, both women and men reported greater intimacy with their best friend than with their romantic partners. When the researchers looked at the kind of factors that were connected to the strength of the relationship, they found that women's friendships depended on the overall closeness of the relationship, including dependability, kindness, and mutual support. In contrast, the strength of men's relationships depended more on how long they had been friends and the social activities they engaged in.[21]

In short, there are general differences between the patterns of women's and men's social relationships. Women tend to have relationships that are closer, more intimate, and depend on mutual support, whereas men's relationships tend to occur around a shared history and shared activities. Given these differences, we can see why women might experience more guilt. For women's friendships, the relationship is more likely to be at risk if one member fails to show appropriate support, caring, or closeness. Experiencing more guilt leads women to express their caring for their friends and bolster the strength of the relationship. However, for men, the shared history and group activities provide more resilience to the relationship. There is less need for men to express their caring for their friends to maintain the health of the relationships, so guilt plays a less important role in relationship management.

The gender differences in guilt-proneness appears to have its origins in family relationships to some extent. Studies that have explored guilt-proneness using the TOSCA and other measures have found that adolescents who report higher levels of closeness to their parents and siblings also report more guilt-proneness. On average, girls report greater closeness to their parents than boys during adolescence, so part of the reason for gender differences in guilt-proneness may be that girls tend to have more intimate family relationships than boys.[22] More generally, across cultures, girls and young women are expected to nurture familial relationships to a greater extent than boys and young men. Such expectations likely have a significant impact on the development of conscience such that, as they develop, women internalize norms associated with maintaining the health of family relationships and, as a consequence, experience greater guilt when they feel that they have not done enough to care for family.

This gender difference in guilt-proneness leads to an interesting possibility concerning the well-established gender difference in delinquency and criminality. Within the general population, there are very strong gender differences in delinquency and criminality, with women much less likely to offend in general than men. Traditional theories of criminality have suggested that differential socialization and role models account for the gender difference in offending. As they develop, boys and men are supposedly more likely to be exposed to models of criminality in their peers and family members, and these patterns rub off on them. But it is also reasonable to suggest that guilt-proneness plays an important role. In fact, there is now good evidence that people who report higher levels of guilt-proneness report lower levels of actual rule-breaking.[23] Recent studies that have compared women's and men's levels of offending have found that the best predictor of differences in offending is guilt-proneness. One recent study examined adolescents' anticipated remorse about shoplifting and found that the amount of guilt reported by girls compared to boys was related to how close they were to their families.[24] So, what we see is that the generally higher guilt-proneness in women compared to men is what may keep them out of trouble to a greater extent!

Cultural Differences in the Experience of Guilt and Shame

So far in this chapter, I have examined how people can be more or less guilt-prone. But it is also possible that different people don't just go through life experiencing more or less guilt; they experience it differently. Back in Chapter 1, I suggested that guilt is a cocktail of fear, sadness, and self-directed anger. Furthermore, when the self-directed anger becomes focused on the self in general and not just on what one has done, guilt morphs into shame. It is generally believed by psychologists that while guilt can be healthy, shame is often unhealthy.[25] Guilt motivates people to repair harms that have been done to others and heal their relationships, whereas shame tends to make people shy away from interpersonal interaction, and so their relationships may remain damaged. But this idea that guilt and shame may play differently in terms of the management of relationships has been brought into question by the study of the experience of guilt and shame in different cultures.

The notion that people in different cultures differ in their experience of guilt and shame in reaction to damaging relationships can be traced to American anthropologist Ruth Benedict's book on Japanese culture, *The Chrysanthemum and the Sword*, published just after the Second World War to help Americans understand their new enemy.[26] In her sweeping survey of politics, business, and family life in Japan, Benedict described how the moral lives of the Japanese were driven more by honor and shame, while Westerners, like citizens of the US, were driven more by guilt. She called Japan a "shame culture" in contrast to the "guilt culture" of the US. This is not to say that guilt has no role in Japanese culture; rather it is that shame plays a different and more prominent role in Japanese culture than in Western cultures.

Benedict pointed out that in contrast to American culture, Japanese culture was very focused on maintaining harmony within the community, which is centered in the family but may extend to society more generally. Benedict's distinction between guilt and shame cultures has become part of the foundation on which a general distinction between what have come to be known as "individualist" and "collectivist" societies has been built.[27] In individualist societies, including most of those in the West, which share a Judeo-Christian heritage and a commitment to liberal-democratic ideology, a person's action tends to be judged according to whether it meets the standards of their individual conscience or the law. In these cultures, both guilt and shame are individual experiences; they differ in terms of whether the person feels bad about what they have done or feels bad about themselves. So, someone is a good person if they act according to their conscience.[28]

In certain collectivist societies, which are more prevalent in Asia and the Middle East, the experience of shame is more common and is tied much more to the group or collective.[29] Someone's action is likely to be judged according to whether it brings honor or shame to their family or community, rather than whether it conforms to the person's individual conscience. The dominant moral code of China, based on the philosophy of Confucius, articulates this idea most clearly. Chinese identity is elaborated in terms of the system of relationships that the person has, whether this be their family or their larger community or workplace. Confucian morality emphasizes the primacy of the family and society over the individual. Everyone's actions are judged in terms of how they maintain or enhance harmony in those social networks or whether they disrupt that harmony. As a result, the experience of guilt and shame is inextricably linked to how actions affect the well-being or harmony of the social network. Shame occurs when someone has failed to uphold the standards of the community, and it depends most importantly on the reactions of that community to what the person has, or has not, done. But, since Confucian morality urges individuals to act to maintain harmony in their social group, shame motivates efforts to maintain or restore such harmony and is seen as a positive emotion.[30] Indeed, shaming is more often used as a parenting strategy by Chinese parents to lead their children to behave in ways that respect the harmony of the social group.[31] As the Chinese philosopher Mencius, perhaps the best-known follower of Confucius, said, "Men cannot live without shame. A sense of shame is the beginning of integrity."[32]

Benedict's work, and the tradition of cross-cultural psychology that followed it, reminds us that the experience of guilt and shame is not necessarily the same across all peoples of the world. Furthermore, research carried out purely on Western populations does not necessarily deliver an understanding of the psychology of guilt and shame that is universally true. Different cultural backgrounds can influence these emotional experiences, and we should always be aware of possible differences among people from different cultures. The difference between individualist and collectivist cultures points to important differences in the ways that guilt and shame may be experienced and acted on. But despite these differences, there are important similarities. Whether people come from more individualist or collectivist cultures, they experience guilt and shame in relation to how they have harmed their relationships. For those in individualist societies, relationships are more likely to be managed in interpersonal ways, so guilt tends to be the dominant emotion.* For those in collectivist cultures, relationships are more strongly conceived in terms of group identity and a network of communal relations. Dishonoring the group results in shame, and it is this shame that helps to guide a person toward appropriate behavior to maintain the harmony within the group as well as the reputation of the group in the eyes of others. So, the role of shame in collectivist cultures is still to manage relationships by restoring the self in the eyes of the group or by restoring the reputation of the group in the eyes of others.

Despite these cultural differences, it's worth noting that there is no hard and fast distinction between guilt and shame cultures. Guilt is still experienced by people in collectivist cultures in the context of harming

---

* In Chapter 11, we will see that there are situations in which people in individualist societies also experience guilt because of harms inflicted by their social group.

another person. Indeed, the Mandarin language has three different words that roughly translate to the English word *guilt*. These three words signify the different layers of guilt that we identified in Chapter 1: the feeling of guilt (*nei jiu*), individual conscience (*zui e gan*), and objective or legal guilt (*fan zui gan*).[33] By the same token, even with the emphasis on individual guilt in Western cultures, it doesn't mean shame in connection with a failure to maintain community harmony is absent. The Western prioritization of guilt over shame is likely a relatively recent phenomenon historically. Certainly, it appears that shame was conceived in more similar ways to contemporary collectivist societies by Western cultures prior to the Enlightenment and the growth of an emphasis on individual rights and freedoms.[34] And it still appears so to some extent today. The shame I felt in connection to my parents after the accident was perhaps a microcosm of shame culture. I grew up in a Western nuclear family, and so I did not experience the pressure from a wider community to meet the standards of the group and maintain community harmony, but certainly there was a hint of what that would be like. I had let my parents down and I felt ashamed of that. In 2016, author David Brooks defended the idea that modern social media platforms such as X and Facebook, limiting as they are for interpersonal interaction, have encouraged a new form of shame culture in the West. Here, in-group collectives of politically like-minded posters pour shame on anyone who dares to post an opinion that deviates from the group party line.[35] So, the difference in the experience of guilt and shame in contemporary individualist and collectivist cultures is really one of degree. While the focus in individualist Western culture tends to be on guilt, in collectivist societies, people's identities are much more bound up in the norms and expectations of their familial and societal networks. Violating these expectations disrupts the harmony of these networks, and feelings of shame may overshadow those of guilt.

Guilt is not just a response to causing harm to a particular relationship at a particular point in time. It is also a general disposition to care about maintaining the health of one's relationships. So, we have looked not just at when and why people feel guilt, but also at who feels guilt. And while guilt is a universal human emotion, not everyone experiences it to the same extent or in the same way. If you are a woman of European heritage living in a Western nation, with a personality that is high on agreeableness, conscientiousness, and neuroticism, then you probably feel a lot of guilt a lot of the time. You care about doing the right thing by others, particularly your many friends, and you work hard to keep your relationships strong. The rest of us also feel guilt, but perhaps not so much and not so often. Is there an optimal level of guilt-proneness? Not at all. It all depends on how much stock you put in ensuring that your network of relationships is healthy. But one thing we can say is that if you almost never feel guilt, then you probably have more trouble keeping relationships. But then you're probably not reading this book!

Part I Takeaways

We know so much more about guilt today than we did when, as a young man, I started to grapple with its meaning in the wake of the accident. Back then, psychology's understanding of guilt was still quite primitive. Guilt was generally seen as a moral emotion dependent on a set of internalized standards for behavior. We have come to see that guilt is, at heart, a response to hurting others with whom we enjoy close relationships, and it serves to protect our most important relationships from the inevitable challenges that arise in everyday social life. The experience of guilt alerts us to the damage that we may have caused to our relationships and goads us into trying to heal those relationships. The experience of guilt urges us to attempt reparation with the victim in an effort to elicit forgiveness from them. In turn, forgiveness resolves guilt by confirming that the relationship remains strong.

A more sophisticated understanding of human emotion has allowed us to see that guilt is not a unique experience. Guilt is a cocktail of other emotions—most importantly, fear or anxiety that a valued relationship has been damaged and may be lost, empathic sadness for the victim, and self-directed anger that takes the form of remorse and regret. These simpler emotions may be mixed in different ways, but two common recipes are "compassionate guilt"—guilt that focuses on the harm suffered by the other—and "remorseful guilt"—guilt that focuses more on self-blame and regret. Compassionate guilt is most likely to motivate reparation and caring for the other. Remorseful guilt tends to lead to self-punishment. Shame, a close emotional cousin of guilt, differs from guilt in that the negative feeling is focused on the self rather than the particular action that has hurt the other, and it is more likely to motivate withdrawal from relationships.

The recognition that guilt builds on simpler emotions in the context of relationship stress has allowed us to recognize that the feeling of guilt can occur in children as young as three years of age. Over time, the guilt that arises in children as their parents attempt to impose compliance around rules for behavior leads to the internalization of rules or standards for behavior. This process of socialization creates the roots of the conscience that each of us carries as our internal guide for good behavior. Parenting styles that encourage empathy for others tend to lead children to experience more compassionate guilt, whereas parenting styles that threaten children with the loss of love or with aggression tend to lead them to experience guilt as remorse or even shame.

Not everyone experiences guilt in the same way or to the same extent: some feel guilt often and in many different circumstances, while others feel guilt rarely or even, in the case of psychopaths, not at all. Those with certain personality styles, including agreeableness, high anxiety, and conscientiousness, tend to report the most guilt. And across cultures, the nature of the relationships that are protected through the experience of guilt varies. Individualist cultures place more emphasis on interpersonal relationships, whereas collectivist cultures may use shame to prioritize the health of the group at the expense of the individual.

We exist in a complicated web of relationships where there is always a chance of hurting those we care about. For the most part, guilt helps to keep our relationships strong, but it can sometimes lead us astray and cause more pain to us than healing of our relationships. So now, let's take a deep dive into the many ways in which guilt appears in our lives.

Part II

Guilt in Everyday Life

Chapter Five

Guilt in Adult Relationships

I still remember quite vividly the first time I felt deeply guilty in a romantic relationship. It was the summer after graduating from high school, and, after a year of trying, I was finally dating the girl I had fallen in love with the moment she walked into my senior biology class. Our plans meant that we were going to be apart for the summer—she on vacation in Spain with her family, and I working close to home to save money for university. One night, our friend group organized a house party, and I found myself talking to another girl I had had a crush on two years earlier but had never dated. She was also seeing someone else who wasn't at the party, but we both knew there was a mutual attraction. We ended up together that night, telling ourselves it was "unfinished business," but making it clear to each other that we were committed to our other relationships. As if it could be so easy! The next day, I was racked by guilt. I had to write a letter to my girlfriend telling her what had happened, apologizing, and telling her it didn't mean anything. In those days before immediate electronic communication, I expected to be languishing in self-reproach and uncertainty for the rest of the summer until she returned from Spain, but within two weeks, a postcard arrived. She told me not to worry; she had been seeing a boy at the resort in Spain, that it was over, and that she was excited to see me soon. Her forgiveness of me and, naturally, my forgiveness of her, dispelled the guilt and strengthened our mutual commitment. We continued to date for another year, until the challenges of maintaining a long-distance relationship—we were at universities in different cities—became too much.

I'm not sure I thought too much about the role of guilt in this episode when it happened, but I still remember well the lessons it taught me. As I reflect back, I think there are two main takeaways. First, no matter how much you love someone, romantic relationships almost always get stress tested at some point or other. The stress may not be as extreme as actual infidelity, although infidelity is not uncommon.[1] But the risk of doing something to hurt your lover at some point in your relationship is almost inevitable, so guilt is a commonplace feature of romance. Second, it is better to take responsibility for your action, own up to your guilt, and seek forgiveness than to deny it. Taking a stance of openness to mutual forgiveness is an important ingredient to a healthy relationship.

Communal and Exchange Relationships

Before we dive into what we know about guilt in adult relationships, take a moment to recall a recent event when you felt really guilty. Was there someone else involved, and if so, what is your relationship with this person?

Every year, when I ask the students in my third year social psychology class to do this exercise, almost without fail, they talk about events involving their close relationships—parents, siblings, romantic partners, friends. My anecdotal research confirms what has been found in more formal studies. In one of the very first published studies to ask people to recall a real-life guilt-laden experience, carried out by Roy Baumeister and his team, over 93 percent of the participants talked about an incident involving a close adult relationship, usually a family member, romantic partner, or close friend.[2]

Within social psychology, these close relationships are known as "communal" relationships. The idea of the communal relationship was first proposed in the late 1970s and studied in detail by two American social psychologists, Margaret Clark and Judson Mills.[3] Prior to their work, social psychologists had mostly studied human interaction by observing how strangers interacted in various situations. Clark and Mills ushered in a new era of studying people in relationships, and they set about trying to distinguish different kinds of relationships. They focused much of their effort on the distinction between two patterns of interaction, which they termed "communal" and "exchange" orientations. These two approaches to relationships both involve partners who are mutually supportive and collaborative, in contrast to relationships that have a competitive or exploitative nature.

Although Clark and Mills make almost no reference in their work to the role of guilt in communal and exchange relationships, I have found their distinction very helpful in thinking about how guilt plays out in our everyday lives. It helps us to understand why we feel more guilt in certain social interactions and relationships, and less or even none in others. The distinction can also help us to understand when the guilt we feel is appropriate, and when and how we should let it go.

In an article reviewing over thirty years of their research, Clark and Mills pose the following question: "Why, when purchasing a gift for a friend, do we expect price tags to be on items yet, after the purchase, we make sure they have been removed?"[4] This question nicely encapsulates the difference between exchange and communal relationships. An exchange relationship, such as the one involved in purchasing an item from a store, is one where interactions primarily involve a sharing or trading of resources or, more generally, "benefits"—anything that one person wants and another can provide. There is a clear and often precise reciprocity. One person provides a benefit to another with the expectation that a benefit of equivalent value will be transferred back within a specified time. When you make a purchase in a store, you provide one form of benefit—money—and you receive a different benefit—some goods or service—in return. Exchange relationships include but go beyond simple economic ones such as purchasing something. In fact, the range of benefits that people provide for each other in exchange relationships is very broad and covers everything from money, food, and objects to personal favors, information, help, and sex. In general, exchange relationships are those where each partner tracks the relative value of the benefits involved to ensure that the outcome is fair.

How each partner in an exchange determines fairness may be highly subjective, and as a result, price setting has become the default way of moderating many exchange relationships, particularly in most westernized societies. But fixed and explicit pricing is a relatively recent and still not universal practice. When I used to visit China on a regular basis to cultivate academic partnerships with Chinese universities, I often went to the Hongqiao, or Pearl, Market in Beijing. The Hongqiao Market is a huge indoor shopping center spread over five floors, with vendor stalls crammed together and selling everything from expensive pearls and jewelry (on the top two floors) to knockoff electronics and "designer" clothing, handbags, and footwear on the bottom two floors. I would go there to buy souvenirs to bring home as gifts for friends and family. There are no marked prices in the Hongqiao Market and bartering is assumed. If you show any interest in their wares, the stall vendors will offer you a price with the expectation that a negotiation will ensue. As a Westerner unused to bartering and having essentially no idea of the true value of most of the items, I started out thinking that I should be aiming for a "sale price" of maybe 25 percent off the price offered. On my first visit, I left with some nice souvenir chopsticks, silk brocade, jade carvings, and the memories of the smiling faces of the vendors. I later realized that those smiling faces meant I had overpaid considerably, and I became annoyed that I had been taken advantage of. On my next trip, I committed to myself that I would not purchase an item unless the vendor had stopped smiling. And sure enough, the harder I bargained, the less happy they became. I still left with some special souvenirs, but the vendors had difficulty suppressing their displeasure. I knew then that I had paid something close to the real value of the items. What was interesting to me in thinking about these purely exchange interactions was that their emotional atmosphere was characterized by the simpler emotions of happiness, disappointment, and anger, but not by guilt or other social emotions. The vendors were happy when they made a good profit and frustrated when they did not. Similarly, I felt happy when I thought I had got the best deal and annoyed when I thought I had been duped. The vendors clearly did not feel guilty when they pressured me into overpaying, and by the same token, I did not feel guilty for pushing as hard as I could for the lowest price—it was just business.

True communal relationships are not like this at all. Communal relationships are dominated by affection and caring for the other. Ideally, relationships between adults are balanced so that each person in the relationship cares for the other equally. There are two sides to communal relationships between adults—loving and being loved. Think about your own communal relationships, perhaps with your romantic partner or, if you don't currently have a romantic partner, your best friend. On the one hand, in loving them, you support their emotional needs. You give them comfort and security in the relationship. You want to look after them and you want them to be happy. In a sense, you act as an attachment figure for them. On the other hand, you also have an attachment to them—you want to stay in close contact with them, you miss them when they are not around, you want to share important aspects of your life experience with them, and so on. Your partner provides for your emotional needs in important ways; they make you feel loved and secure in the comfort of the relationship. Communal relationships between adults, such as romantic relationships and friendships tend to be symmetrical in the sense that the relationship is built on both partners caring for each other.

In communal relationships, caring is provided when it is needed, not based on whether the partner is able to reciprocate. While there may be an expectation of mutual caring, a strict tally of the benefits provided is not kept. Indeed, in some communal relationships, the caring may be largely one-way or asymmetrical. Parents care for their dependent children in multiple ways with little expectation of caring in return. Benefits largely flow in one direction—from parent to child. Of course, children also care deeply about their parents and show this caring through their affection. So, it is not as though there are no benefits to being a parent. This one-way transfer of benefits may switch later in life as an aging parent becomes dependent on their child for care. And families provide the context for most cases of asymmetrical communal relationships. For example, someone with a significant physical or mental disability will, in most cases, receive substantial care from family members, whether they be parents, spouses, or siblings. We will explore some of these patterns of asymmetrical communal relationships and the guilt that characterizes them in the following two chapters.

So, in communal relationships, you care about the interests and emotional needs of the other, and fairness is not a priority or perhaps even a consideration. And that is why we do not want our gifts to friends to reveal their cost. To do so would lead to an implicit expectation that the recipient owes us something of equal value, and it would tilt the relationship from a communal one to one of exchange.

The pattern of mutual caring in communal relationships involves a different set of emotions than exchange relationships. We provide benefits to communal partners because we feel affection for them. We empathically feel their distress if they are somehow upset, we get sad if they neglect or harm us, and we feel guilty when we hurt them in some way or fail to provide the attention, caring, and support they need. Guilt plays an especially important role in communal relationships, because it orients us to keeping these relationships healthy.

While some relationships are clearly primarily communal, such as between romantic partners, and some are clearly primarily exchange, such as between customer and shopkeeper, many relationships may be communal or exchange at root but have, or acquire, features of the other type. Perhaps you had a favorite local restaurant that was imperiled during the Covid-19 pandemic restrictions, and you gave extra-large tips when you ordered their take-out food. In this case, while the relationship between you and the restaurant owner was essentially one of exchange, you gave a bit extra because you cared about the restaurant owner, not only because they provided you with good food for your money, but also because they were part of your community. Or perhaps you share an apartment with a close friend. You each care for the other in a communal way, but you also have an arrangement where you both share the apartment expenses equally and keep a tally of who has paid for what. So, it is perhaps better to think of most relationships as having some balance of communal and exchange elements. However, the more we interact with someone, the greater the likelihood that the relationship will acquire communal features and the greater the likelihood we will feel guilty when we do something that threatens the relationship.

The other point to make about the difference between communal and exchange relationships is that the particular individuals in the former group are relatively fixed, whereas those in the latter group can be easily swapped out and vary much more over time. We care in a communal way about certain people—members of our family, friends, and so on—and we typically maintain these relationships over long periods of time. But we can engage with anyone using exchange norms. It does not matter if the shop assistant helping me today is a different person from the one who helped me yesterday; my interaction can still follow the same exchange norm.

Of course, we all know that we can and do feel guilt in connection with mere acquaintances and even strangers. Sometimes, this guilt may arise because we are in a role that carries with it a responsibility of care and we fail in that responsibility. By far the most heartbreaking personal example of guilt that has been brought up in my social psychology class over the years was from a student who was a lifeguard at a public swimming pool. He recounted how he had failed to save a young child from drowning and had been preoccupied with guilt ever since. Guilt also comes from the sense of obligation provided by our conscience. Encountering a homeless person on the street may incline us to give them some money, and perhaps we feel a twinge of guilt if we do not. Here, the guilt arises not from any relationship with the homeless person, but from the expectations we have for our own good behavior. But overall, these kinds of guilt-inducing events are much less frequent in day-to-day life than those involving our communal relationships.

We also find that while everyone has some relationships that are primarily communal and others that are primarily exchange, people differ to the extent that they believe that relationships should be communal or exchange in general. Margaret Clark's research group has developed brief questionnaires to assess what they call "communal orientation" and "exchange orientation."[5] Overall, their research has shown that having a communal orientation to family members is relatively universal, but the extent to which people have communal orientations to those who are not family varies considerably. People who have a high communal orientation are more likely than those with low communal orientation to help a stranger in need, particularly if that person seems sad.[6] With these facts in mind, think back to Chapter 4, where we explored the idea of "guilt-proneness," or the idea that some people experience more guilt than others. It should come as no surprise that people who tend to be very communally oriented also tend to be guilt-prone.[7]

Some psychologists believe that the most prominent communal relationships between adults—including the ones with romantic partners and even close friends—all link back to the relationship bonds that characterize extended family groups.[8] And, the family relationships that we all experience growing up impact, to some extent, the way we manage our adult communal relationships. Communal relationships involving relatively selfless caring for others are inherent in families. Because family members are usually genetically related or, in the case of romantic partners, are tied together through their shared contribution to their children, who are genetically related, selfless caring for family members, or "kin" to use the more formal term, is adaptive from an evolutionary point of view. As a result, the psychology that supports selfless caring, including emotions like guilt, is most obvious among kin. But this psychology can also take root in relationships between unrelated people, most notably close friends. So, let's explore how these other strong relationships become established, and how guilt plays its part in forging them and, sometimes, breaking them apart.

Lovers

Most people invest a lot of time, energy, and, of course, money in trying to secure and keep healthy and fulfilling romantic relationships. As a general rule, the more satisfied people are with their romantic relationships, the more they report overall happiness and life satisfaction.[9] And for most people, a communal approach to such relationships is preferable to an exchange approach.[10] That's not to say there won't be exchange elements to these relationships—couples may negotiate between them a fair distribution of chores and expenses—and those exchange elements may contribute to relationship satisfaction. But the overall quality of satisfying romantic relationships is maintained through affection and caring for the partner.

Although romantic relationships occur between people who are not closely related genetically, they assume the status of kin relations. In fact, it is quite well-established that they carry echoes of the attachment relationship between child and parent. As is quite well-known, Freud believed that the psychosexual development of boys and girls grows out of their relationships with their parents.[11] In more modern research, the notion that early child-parent attachment relationships provide a basis for adult romantic relationships has gained significant support. John Bowlby, the psychologist we met in Chapter 3 who originated modern attachment theory, argued that the patterns of attachment between children and their parents established in early infancy go on to influence how people develop loving relationships in adulthood.[12] The core idea that explains the link between early attachment relationships between children and their parents and romantic attachments in adults is that of the "internal working model." As children, we develop expectations about the ways our parents respond to our needs, particularly our needs for love and security. When there is a good fit between a child's needs and the parent's response, the child develops a set of expectations— the internal working model—that intimate relationship partners are emotionally sensitive and reliable. This is the "secure" attachment style that we encountered in Chapter 3. Where the fit is less good, the child may develop an insecure attachment style for which the internal working model is that the intimate partner is less emotionally sensitive and reliable. These internal working models influence how we behave as adults in intimate relationships and guide both the choice of partner and the ways we interact with that partner.

Social psychologists Cindy Hazan and Phillip Shaver were the first to study whether adult romantic relationships to some extent mirror those established in early childhood.[13] In their influential work, they collaborated with a newspaper to recruit adults to respond to a questionnaire about the "love of your life." The questionnaire asked respondents to answer a set of questions about their experience of romantic relationships. For one important question, respondents rated themselves according to three "adult attachment types," which were constructed based on the types of attachment relationships seen in young children. Read the descriptions below and, while reflecting on your own intimate relationships, think about which fits you best. If you have a significant other at this time, think about what category would fit them best as well.

> 1. I find it relatively easy to get close to others and am comfortable depending on them and having them depend on me. I don't worry about being abandoned or about someone getting too close to me.
>
> 2. I am somewhat uncomfortable being close to others; I find it difficult to trust them completely, difficult to allow myself to depend on them. I am nervous when anyone gets too close, and often, love partners want me to be more intimate than I feel comfortable being.
>
> 3. I find that others are reluctant to get as close as I would like. I often worry that my partner doesn't really love me or won't stay with me. I want to merge completely with another person, and this desire sometimes scares people away.

Of nearly six hundred respondents across a wide age range, about 56 percent rated themselves as closest to the first type, which is called the "secure" type following the research on attachment in children.

Some 25 percent rated themselves in the second group, which is the "avoidant" type, and about 19 percent rated themselves as the third "anxious" type. Interestingly, these proportions correspond closely to the proportions of these attachment types seen in young children. When Hazan and Shaver asked their participants to describe their relationships as children with their parents, adults with secure attachments reported having more affectionate, caring parents, whereas adults with anxious or avoidant attachments described relationships with their own parents that were more distant, unpredictable, or rejecting. This correspondence suggests, but of course by no means proves, that adult romantic attachment styles are related to those seen in early childhood toward parents.

We know from studies of people in romantic relationships, from dating to marriage, that attachment style is connected to relationship longevity and satisfaction. Those who are secure in their attachment style report higher satisfaction with their romantic relationships overall than those who are insecure—both anxious and avoidant.[14] They describe their relationships as more loving, passionate, intimate, and committed. They also report that both they and their partner carry out selfless acts to meet the needs of the other. This difference in relationship satisfaction translates into different prospects for relationship success. In general, those who are securely attached show greater commitment to their relationships, which last longer and are less likely to end in breakup or divorce, compared to those who show an insecure attachment style.

But that doesn't mean that the romantic relationships of securely attached people are free of the challenges created by one or the other partner doing something to hurt the other. The critical issue is how people with different attachment styles respond to these challenges, and here, guilt appears to play an important role. Those who are secure in their attachment style tend to experience guilt when they have done something to upset their partner. And then they are likely to act on their guilt by seeking forgiveness from their partner through apology or doing something for their partner by way of reparation. In this way, the health of the relationship becomes quickly restored.

Surprisingly, only a few studies have explicitly examined guilt in relation to the different styles of romantic attachment, but they reveal a consistent story. Frederick Lopez and his colleagues were the first to directly examine people's attachment styles and their experience of guilt and shame in their relationships.[15] They measured the degree to which their participants experienced both avoidance and anxiety in their relationships. They also tested them on the TOSCA measure of guilt- and shame-proneness.[16] They found that avoidance was related to guilt-proneness such that the *more* avoidant people were, the *less* they appeared to experience guilt in their relationships. This pattern shows that guilt is connected to being invested in the relationship; if you avoid intimacy, then you experience less guilt. In contrast, anxiety was more related to shame-proneness—people who reported more anxiety in their relationships also reported more shame. Those who tend to be anxious in their relationships view themselves as relatively unlovable, and so when they do something that might harm their relationship, it reinforces this negative sense of self. Those who fit the core pattern of secure attachment—low avoidance and low anxiety—experience guilt rather than shame, which leads them to try to heal their relationships when they have been tested.

A subsequent study by the team led by Phillip Shaver added an assessment of hostility in addition to guilt and shame.[17] The researchers asked participants to report their levels of anxiety and avoidance in their intimate relationships, and then asked them to recall and write about an episode when they had hurt their romantic partner in some way or failed to meet their romantic partner's needs. After writing about the episode, the participants were asked to rate the extent to which remembering the episode made them feel guilt, shame, and anger. In line with the earlier study, attachment anxiety was strongly related to shame—those who reported more relationship anxiety also reported more shame. Also in agreement with the earlier study, attachment avoidance was negatively associated with guilt and shame in connection with the recalled event. What was new was that those high in attachment avoidance reported significantly more hostility toward their aggrieved partner than those low in avoidance.

This finding that people who are avoidant in relationships experience hostility rather than guilt when they have done something to upset their relationship partner brings us back to the difference between communal and exchange orientations. Recall that guilt occurs in those who adopt a communal approach to a relationship, whereas anger tends to be associated with an exchange approach, particularly if there is a sense that reciprocity and fairness have not been achieved. The difference in emotional reaction to a relationship partner being upset suggests that whereas securely and anxiously attached people tend to assume a communal approach to their relationships, avoidantly attached people tend to treat their relationships on more of an exchange basis.

This issue has been studied explicitly by Jennifer Bartz and John Lydon at McGill University.[18] They asked people who were secure, anxious, or avoidant in their romantic relationships to rate how they would feel in response to caring (or communal) situations. These situations included a partner unexpectedly paying for their dinner and a partner asking for emotional support. Those who were secure generally responded positively to these partner caring situations—they were happy to both receive care from and provide care for their partner—and they were unconcerned about reciprocation from the other or for the other's caring acts. The anxious participants were happy to receive and provide care, but these situations also made them stressed, and they expressed concern about whether their partner might reciprocate when they had provided care for their partner. Finally, the participants who were avoidant were less keen about receiving an unsolicited act of caring from their partner and about responding to the other's needs. They expressed both anxiety and considerable annoyance in reaction to these communal episodes. They wanted to be able to reciprocate quickly when their partner did something for them to discharge the debt, and they also expressed more concern about whether their own acts of caring would be reciprocated. These findings suggest that whereas securely and anxiously attached people tend to follow communal norms in their relationships, avoidantly attached people are more likely to adopt exchange norms.

An intriguing implication of this difference in approach to relationships is that those who are avoidantly attached are more likely to engage in infidelity. Earlier, we saw that communal relationships are with particular people whom we care about, whereas exchange relationships are less dependent upon any particular individual. If one carries an exchange orientation into one's romantic relationships, then one will tend to be less committed to one's partner. Studies of partner commitment, infidelity, and relationship breakups have shown that avoidantly attached people are less committed to their partners than securely and anxiously attached people, and that this lower commitment leads them to expect that their relationships will not work out in the long run and to be more likely to engage in extra-relationship affairs.[19] It seems, then, that the reduced guilt experienced by avoidant partners results in a far greater likelihood of relationship failure.

When we put all of these findings together, we see that attachment style, communal or exchange orientation, and the experience of guilt all interact to affect the health of romantic relationships. The model for healthy close relationships appears to be one where both partners tend to have a communal orientation and a secure attachment style. Under these circumstances, guilt tends to arise naturally when the relationship is threatened, and it leads both partners to increase their caring for the other, securing their bond.

Friends

I have to admit, I'm not terribly good at friendships. Like most introverts, if there's a choice between staying home and reading a book or going out for dinner with friends, I'll usually prefer to stay home. My circle of friends is small, and they are mostly people with whom I share a passion, usually connected to my intellectual and academic pursuits or sports. Much of my social life is organized through my wife, a not unusual circumstance for older married men. Sometimes, I worry that my neglect of friendships will come back to haunt me. As Marisa Franco shows in her book *Platonic*,[20] people with a healthy circle of close friends tend to have higher life satisfaction, be healthier, and even live longer. But despite being a bit stunted on the friendship front, I think I have a pretty clear sense of what it means to be, or have, a close friend.

To my mind, having a close friend is the purest kind of symmetrical communal relationship. Friends care for each other simply because they value the relationship. As we shall see in the next two chapters, parent-child relationships are not symmetrical. One member of the relationship does most of the heavy lifting in terms of caring—the parent when the child is young and, often, the child when the parent is old. Romantic relationships are ideally symmetrical, certainly at first. Indeed, the most recent research on pathways to romance suggests that friendship-based intimacy is more common than, and preferred to, passion-based intimacy in the formation of both cross-gender and same-gender romantic relationships.[21] But long-lasting romantic relationships often become organized around children, and with that, their communal focus can become consumed with caring for the children rather than each other.

In the modern era of Facebook friendships often numbering in the many hundreds or even thousands, it is interesting to consider who of all the people we may know really counts as a friend. A reasonable criterion (if not definition) is that a friend is someone who is unrelated to us by blood or marriage but with whom we share a communal relationship to some degree. Robin Dunbar, who has spent a lifetime studying friendships and whose work we briefly reviewed in Chapter 4, suggests that friends are "the people you wouldn't feel embarrassed about asking for a favor and whom you wouldn't think twice about helping out."[22]

Dunbar and his collaborators have shown through various ingenious approaches that the approximate size limit of the circle of people with whom we have a communal relationship is 150, which has come to be known as "Dunbar's number."[23] This is the approximate group size that humans are able to keep track of. Many of the people in this group will be kin, but Dunbar suggests that after extended family, there is still room for a stock of unrelated people with whom we share communal relations. In this approach to friendship, friends include both relatives and unrelated people, so Dunbar's number essentially captures the group of people with whom someone enjoys some degree of communal relationship.

The evidence for Dunbar's number is extensive and comes from sources as diverse as the average number of people invited to a wedding in the US, the average number of people on a British Christmas card list during the 1990s, and the average number of people called in a year, not counting businesses, determined by an analysis of cell phone records. Dunbar's number is not just a feature of friendship circles of modern Western life. Dunbar and his colleagues examined typical community sizes of hunter-gatherer and traditional horticulturalist societies and found that they included, on average, about 150 people. This was also the approximate size of the population of medieval villages in England as reported in the Domesday Book, the first complete census of a country, carried out by William the Conqueror in 1086 AD. Even today, more traditionally structured communities in the West seem to conform to

Dunbar's number. For example, North American Hutterite farming colonies, which are organized around a communal, mutually supportive lifestyle, fission into two communities when the overall group size grows too large. A review of such fissions suggests that they occur, on average, when the parent colony reaches around 150 members.[24]

One interesting implication of Dunbar's work is that having a large group of friends in the sense that we understand the term—unrelated people with whom we share a communal relationship—is a relatively recent development historically and culturally. Traditionally, communal groups were made up primarily of relatives by blood and by marriage. Dunbar suggests that we all have a relatively fixed number of communal positions, and relatives fill them up first, but those left over become available for unrelated people whom we care about.[25] These days, at least in the West, our extended families tend to be smaller, and so our communities include a broad range of people, who may be widely geographically dispersed, with whom we share common activities, including work and recreation. But even today, relatives take priority in our allocation of caring. People who come from large extended families tend to have a smaller number of unrelated friends than people who come from smaller families. Unrelated friends assume quasi-familial status, and we care for them and about them in a similar way as we do for family. We can observe this in the way we commonly adopt kinship labels to describe our friends, for example, we use "bro" and "sister" as terms of affection for our close friends, or we might refer to a close family friend as "Auntie Jo" or "Uncle Jim." Nevertheless, as the old saying goes, blood is thicker than water.

People sometimes object to Dunbar's number because they think about the size of their closest friend group, which is much smaller, or the number of "friends" they have on social media platforms such as Facebook, which is often much larger. The group of 150 is really the rough size of the community that one person can keep on top of in terms of tracking who is who, what their role in the larger community is, and to whom the person feels some degree of communal orientation. But within this community, individuals will also engage with smaller circles of friends, most notably a small group of about five close friends, who are the ones you interact with frequently and rely on for emotional support, and a slightly larger group of people of about fifteen who socialize together relatively often and with whom communal norms are predominant. These friend circles reflect degrees of communality. The few people within the inner circle are those who are, or who most resemble, immediate family. These are the friendships that we care most about and, by the same token, are most prone to producing guilt.

What is the role of guilt in friendships? As for all communal relationships, we feel guilt in friendships when we have done, or perhaps think we have done, something to harm the relationships with our friend. Think back to the example of gossiping that we explored in Chapter 2. In that case, the guilt served to focus attention on the threat to the relationship and motivated the attempt to rectify the harm. When we hurt a friend and feel bad about it, apology and, hopefully, forgiveness from the friend allow us to reclaim the health of the relationship.

As with other communal relationships, attachment style can influence how people engage in friendships. When it comes to friendships, the original attachment style developed in the child-parent relationship may have only limited impact. While there is some consistency in people's attachment style in relation to parents, to romantic partners, and to friends, there is also a lot of variation across relationships.[26] One's attachment orientation with a friend also depends importantly on the friend's orientation. So, we should not assume that people who start out with a more secure, anxious, or avoidant attachment style with their parents will automatically translate these styles into how they interact with friends. Sometimes, being secure, anxious, or avoidant in a friendship may be a reaction to that particular relationship. Nevertheless, the style of relating to others will impact the relationship orientation. There is almost no research on how people with different friend attachment styles show guilt, but it is reasonable to expect that friendship attachment dynamics will have similar effects on how guilt is used in friendship management as we see in romantic relationships. If you are relatively secure in a friendship, then you will likely enjoy a mutually communal orientation within the relationship. You may let your friend down once in a while, but you will likely feel some guilt about that and try to make it up to them. If you are anxious in a friendship, you may be overly concerned that your friendship is always at risk. You may treat any suggestions of coolness from your friend as a sign that they don't care for you and that you are unlovable. This anxiety may lead you to seek constant signals from your friend that you are loved—an approach that can be off-putting if, as we will see later in the chapter, it involves guilt-tripping—or to withdraw in shame and anger from the friendship altogether. Finally, for those with a more avoidant style, it is likely that the relationship will be treated with more of an exchange than a communal orientation and guilt will be less in play.

There are two additional points worth making on friendships and guilt. The first is that friends are the earliest relationships that are genuinely symmetrical. As they establish friendships within peer groups at school or in recreational activities, children encounter situations with their friends where they may fail to care for others and where others hurt them. They enjoy the rewards of sharing activities and experiences with their friends, and suffer the empathic sadness and remorse that comes with hurting a friend. And they get the pleasure of being supported by their friends as well as the pain from sometimes being hurt by them. Friendships are the crucible in which a genuinely communal approach to relationships is first forged. To that point, a lot of research has shown that one of the key ingredients of guilt—empathy—is facilitated by having close friends. Indeed, it is likely that friends are more important for the development of empathy in childhood than are parents.[27]

The second point is that friendships can provide a buffering of the experience of guilt. We have seen how guilt comes not only from the threat to the relationship with someone we have harmed directly, but also from the fear of how others in a peer group may view us. The value of a good friend in this context is to provide support and validation. Thinking back again to our gossiping example, let's imagine you apologized to your friend after gossiping about them, but they were reluctant to forgive you, leaving your guilt to fester. If other close friends in your peer group recognize your genuine attempt at reconciliation, respect you for it, and believe you deserve forgiveness, then a kind of vicarious forgiveness can be achieved. When I was suffering from guilt in the aftermath of the accident, the support of my friends certainly contributed to the relief I was able to attain. Such an environment of forgiveness from friends can go a long way to relieving one's guilt.

Siblings

Sibling relationships present another different context for the experience of guilt. For those of us who have them, siblings are often our most enduring communal relationships, longer than our relationships with our parents, our spouses, and our friends. Siblings are our closest kin, with whom we share heritage and history. For many of us, our siblings are also some of our closest adult supporters and confidants. But we do not get to choose our siblings, unlike our romantic partners and friends; we are thrust together in the environment of the family, and it is in this setting that sibling relationships are first forged and sometimes broken.

I have suggested that caring communal relationships are most prominent in families. But a communal orientation is not always the way that siblings view each other, especially when young. Many years ago, child psychiatrist David Levy coined the term "sibling rivalry" to denote the jealousy and hostility that are commonly experienced by older children across cultures in reaction to the arrival of a younger sibling, especially if they are close in age.[28] Within the family context, competition among siblings during childhood often arises naturally as they vie with each other for parental attention and resources. Throughout the animal world, the degree to which parents are able to care for their offspring is limited, and so offspring will often compete for what's available. Siblicide may occur in animals when food is in short supply. For example, in birds, stronger nestlings will sometimes dump their weaker siblings out of the nest.[29] Notwithstanding the biblical story of Cain and Abel, siblicide is rare in humans. However, particularly when children are close in age, competition between siblings can be fierce. Older, particularly male, siblings often attempt to exert their dominance, and bullying is not uncommon.[30]

I experienced this dynamic firsthand growing up as the middle child of three for the first ten years of my life. When we were both of preschool age, I was enamored of my sister, who was a mere eighteen months younger than me, and the roots of a strong communal relationship were established. I remember asking my father to take me to the library when I was four, so I could get a book to read for her. A photo from that day shows my sister in her crib with me next to her, holding a copy of *Little Red Riding Hood*. But I can also remember vividly the oppressive presence of my sister through my childhood as we grew older. She was much cuter and more charming than me, and, before long, she became more athletic than me. I feared that she would displace me in my parents' affections, and this feeling persisted into early adolescence. At its height, I can only describe the experience as a feeling of dread of impending annihilation.

This anxiety made me resent her, and too often, I'm embarrassed to admit, I took it out on her. I would not say that I was a bully in the sense of aggressively targeting her in a sustained way, but when we would get into conflict, I was not shy about using physical force and doing my best to make her cry. I don't remember feeling any guilt as a child about the way I treated my sister. As we grew into middle childhood, the competitive side of our relationship became dominant, and there was little or no communal nature to our relationship. But as I matured through adolescence and transitioned away from the family, our relationship evolved into one of friendship and mutual caring. When I looked back as an adult on the way I had behaved toward her when we were children, I certainly felt guilt. In time, that guilt began to cast a shadow over how I saw our relationship, and I finally apologized for how I had treated her when we were children. Now, over sixty years later from when we first "met," we remain very close.

Unfortunately, however, sustained sibling bullying during childhood can overwhelm and destroy any communal orientation, and it is, perhaps, the most common reason why sibling relationships break down completely. As Louise, who was a respondent to a BBC News story[31] on sibling bullying, reported:

> We bullied each other very badly. I had aggressive physical fights with my brother all the way into our mid-teens. He told me I was fat and ugly until after I left home and dropped to six stone, when he seemed to realise the effect of his words and wouldn't shut up about how thin I was. I was scared of him physically and so I made comments to try and dent his confidence. I suppose it was a self-perpetuating circle of his physically punishing me for my comments and me making comments to punish him for physically beating me.

> For my part, I said some absolutely unforgiveable things to him which even as an adult I feel incapable of repeating because I still feel so ashamed. My brother and I now have very little contact. He's struggling with life and has struggled with drug problems, relationship and mental health issues. I feel responsible for this, and I don't think I'll ever be able to let that guilt go but I don't know how to apologise or make up for the things I said and did.

The guilt that Louise feels reveals that her relationship with her brother is still meaningful to her. But unfortunately, their shared history of conflict has so damaged their relationship that the guilt cannot do its work in motivating mutual forgiveness. Fortunately, in most cases, sibling conflict does not inevitably end in relationship breakdown. Even in cases where the early conflict was destructive, guilt, apology, and forgiveness can go a long way to restoring the relationship.

Is there anything that parents can do to ease the early development of the sibling relationship along a more communal path? In her landmark study of the development of sibling relationships, British psychologist Judy Dunn noted that the stronger the relationship between parent and firstborn, the more likely it was that the firstborn would show ambivalent or outright aggressive behavior toward a younger sibling.[32] And in time, not surprisingly, the younger sibling would become more negative toward the older child. This dynamic discourages the development of a communal relationship between the siblings and can lead to mutual antagonism during childhood. Later in life, both siblings may feel retrospective guilt, but at that point, it may be more difficult to resolve. Dunn found that those parents who involved the older sibling directly in the care of the younger sibling, not as a chore but as something they could do together, encouraged a more positive attitude in their older children toward their younger sibling. Caring for the younger child became a joint activity and a way of bonding for the parent and older child. Over time, this dynamic played out with the older child becoming much more affectionate toward the younger, who, in turn, became more positive toward the older sibling. And, in this way, a mutually communal relationship between the siblings developed from an early age. There are important lessons in this work:

relationship management often involves multiple intersecting relationships, and nowhere is this more true than within the family. Siblings that learn to care for each other from a young age develop a strong communal relationship in which guilt, when it occurs, can help manage the relationship in a healthy way throughout life.

Guilt-Tripping

So far in this chapter, we have looked at a variety of communal relationships, and I have argued throughout that guilt is a powerful emotional force that, within the context of a relationship, motivates a person to try to keep that relationship healthy. Guilt is not just a feeling; it is a call to action. This motivational aspect of guilt creates the opportunity for one partner in a relationship to influence the other by making them feel guilty. And so, we see the possibility for what is sometimes called the "guilt trip," whereby one partner intentionally makes the other feel guilty to get them to act in a certain way.

In psychology, the guilt trip is known more prosaically as "guilt induction." We introduced this idea in Chapter 3 when we talked about parenting strategies. In their efforts to mold their children's behavior to conform to social norms, parents often aim, either intentionally or not, to make their children feel guilty about what they have done. Perhaps the clearest example is how parents encourage prosocial behavior, such as fairness, helpfulness, or caring for others, rather than antisocial behavior, such as selfishness or aggression. Parents often try to elicit empathy in their children by drawing their attention to the harm that has been caused to someone else. The point is to help the child learn that certain ways of behaving are socially inappropriate or harmful to others, so that they won't be inclined to act that way again. This kind of parental guilt induction is generally done for the good of the child, so one might think of it as a form of education. The parent benefits, of course, by having a child who is well-behaved, but the real purpose is to educate the child in the ways of the social world.

Within adult relationships, guilt induction is rarely done by one person for the benefit of the other. It is done as an indirect way to get the other to do something that will be of benefit to oneself. In perhaps the first systematic study of guilt induction in adults, Anita

Vangelisti and her colleagues at the University of Texas asked adults to report conversations in which either they had made someone else feel guilty or another person had made them feel guilty.[33] They also asked their participants to rate how close they were to the other person. It was revealing that the participants found it very easy to report guilt-inducing conversations, both where they had induced guilt in the other and where the other had induced guilt in them, suggesting that these were common occurrences. The conversations were almost all with people to whom they were very close, such as family, spouses, and good friends. Guilt induction very rarely occurred between strangers. The most common guilt conversations involved an attempt to persuade the other to do something. Inducing guilt for persuasion benefits the guilt inducer by harnessing the power of guilt to convince the other to do something that the guilt inducer wants done. Here's an example from the study in which a mother attempts to persuade her spouse to watch their child by pointing out how he is failing to live up to the expectations of his role as a father. The mother induces guilt by suggesting a threat to the developing relationship between the father and his son:

> Mother: Are you going to watch the baby tomorrow while I'm in school?
>
> Father: No, I want to go fishing.
>
> Mother: Fine. When he grows up and asks who Daddy is, I'll say he never had time for you.

Vangelisti and her colleagues also found that people who use guilt-induction tactics in this way tend to be less assertive in general. This kind of persuasion tactic takes the place of more direct forms of coercion, including overt aggression. In this way, guilt induction provides a tool for those who are less assertive to get their way without appearing overtly demanding.

So far, we have outlined two ways in which people use guilt induction—for education and for persuasion. There is a third use of guilt induction, which is more commonly associated with the idea of the guilt trip, and that is to manage one's relationship with another person.

In a study like the one carried out by Vangelisti and colleagues, Roy Baumeister's team asked participants to write a description of an event in which they had made someone else feel guilty or someone else had made them feel guilty.[34] Again, almost all these events happened between people in close relationships, such as parents and children or romantic partners. In this study, the most common reason for inducing guilt was feeling neglected, such as one person feeling that their relationship partner was not spending enough time with them or paying enough attention to them.

When it comes to romantic relationships, guilt induction is a common tool to elicit signals of love and commitment from the partner. Having read earlier about the different styles of romantic attachment, you may not be surprised to learn that guilt induction is not used equally by people with different attachment styles. Anxiously attached people are constantly vigilant for the signals of love and commitment from their partners that will allow them to feel secure in their relationship. A very common way to elicit these signals is to make their partners feel guilty, so that those partners will demonstrate their commitment to the relationship. Studies of the guilt-induction tactics employed by anxiously attached people include using, and often exaggerating, emotional expressions conveying hurt, such as sulking and pouting, appealing for expressions of love and commitment from the partner, presenting the self as needy, and claiming to be hurt by the partner's actions. All these tactics invite the partner to show that they care.

Nickola Overall and her research team at the University of Auckland in New Zealand have studied this emotional dynamic in depth. In one of their studies, they recruited a sample of 180 heterosexual couples, who had been together for at least a year, to enroll in a study of relationship satisfaction.[35] At the outset of the study, each member of the couple completed a rating of their attachment style to assess both anxiety and avoidance in relationships. They also gave an assessment of their overall satisfaction with their relationship. Then, they were engaged in a conversation together about the one thing each would want to change about the other. The point of this part of the study was to introduce a stressor into the relationship to see to what extent guilt induction would emerge as a tactic. To measure guilt induction, the researchers coded the couples' conversations for a range of different tactics such as exaggerated expressions, like pouting, indicating hurt, or portraying themselves as more in need of help or support. Following this conversation, each member of the couple rated their feelings during the conversations, focusing on how angry, hurt, and guilty they felt. Finally, there were follow-ups every three months for a year for which the participants reported on their overall relationship satisfaction.

The findings showed that people who are more anxiously attached are more hurt by relationship stress, and they respond to this stress by engaging in more guilt-induction tactics than those who are less anxiously attached. Further, the partners of those high-anxiety individuals sense this greater hurt, and they themselves feel guiltier than partners of low-anxiety individuals. As the relationship continues, there appear to be consequences of this guilt dynamic. Anxiously attached people who had partners who experienced more guilt reported better relationship satisfaction in the follow-up phase of the study. However, the partners of these highly anxious people who expressed more hurt and induced more guilt ended up reporting lower relationship satisfaction during the follow-up phase. As Overall and her colleagues concluded, "Ironically, the strategies that help anxious individuals obtain the reassurance they need also increases the long-term risk of the rejection they ultimately fear."[36]

Guilt induction in romantic relationships seems to be a particularly common tactic for people who have an anxious attachment style. As a relationship management tactic, it may be effective within reason for getting one's partner to amplify their caring. But too much guilt induction seems not to be effective, and it can lead to a certain amount of resentment from their partner. After all, who wants to be made to feel continuously guilty by one's partner for not caring enough? It can also backfire when the partner tends to have an avoidant attachment style. If the purpose of guilt induction is to increase intimacy and caring behavior from one's partner, then we can see that it might be particularly counterproductive when the partner prefers not to be intimate. And this is what Nickola Overall's team found. Relationship satisfaction is especially poor in couples where one partner has an anxious attachment style and engages in guilt induction with their partner who has an avoidant attachment style. This combination of styles is markedly incompatible and does not bode well for the long-term success of the relationship.

No relationships are smooth sailing all the way. Communal relationships between adults, whether lovers, friends, or siblings are regularly tinged with guilt. These relationships are founded on caring for each other, but that doesn't mean that one person in the relationships will not from time to time do something to hurt the other. The guilt that follows may make us feel bad, but it is toward a noble end. It reflects the value that we place in those we care about. When we feel guilt, we are more likely to work to restore relationship harmony. Indeed, guilt is perhaps the most important psychological mechanism that we have for keeping these mutually rewarding relationships healthy.

In this chapter, we have focused on relationships that ideally have a symmetrical and reciprocal nature. Next, we turn to communal relationships where one partner is doing most of the work in caring for the other. In these relationships, guilt tends to be concentrated in the carer, and, as we will see, the demands of caring combined with the quality of the relationship are significant factors in determining how that guilt is experienced. In the next chapter, we will look at the experience of parenthood and the part that guilt plays in fulfilling that responsibility.

Chapter Six

Parental Guilt

"She's a little piranha," the maternity ward nurse said as our day-old daughter gummed aggressively at Shannon's breast. "It's common—some babies take a while to latch on; just see how it goes."[1] Shannon smiled confidently at the nurse and turned back to trying to arrange Mackenzie's mouth around her nipple. Feeling rather useless, I smiled encouragingly and left them to it. We had been through the antenatal program and were confident she would get the hang of it soon. The amusing image of my newborn daughter as a voracious carnivorous fish played in my head as I watched them.

Three weeks later, Shannon was sitting up in our bed, crying from pain and frustration. Her nightgown hung loose to reveal her cracked and swollen left nipple, the areola of which was starting to detach from her breast in one place. She tried to cradle our daughter, who was tense and crying loudly from hunger. Mackenzie had managed to take an ounce or two of milk over the last few hours, but it had been a long struggle for both of them. Try as they might, they could not find a consistent connection between mouth and nipple. The last three weeks had been just like this, and they both appeared defeated. I stood by, available but impotent; this was their challenge to work through. Finally, Shannon looked toward me, tears flowing, and we knew what we had to do. I left immediately and drove to the drugstore. Thirty minutes later, our daughter was cradled warmly in her mother's arms and sucking contentedly on a bottle of formula.

When Shannon recalls this event, she remembers the pain of mastitis and the frustration of trying with such limited success to breastfeed. But she also recalls sadness and guilt that she could not establish this most intimate of connections with her baby: "I so desperately wanted to continue to nourish her from my body on the outside just as I had for nine months on the inside. Even though I knew it was a problem with the latch, I still felt that I had let her down by not being able to provide this emotional connection for her, and that guilt stayed with me for some time."

Guilt is a regular emotional experience for parents. It comes often and for all sorts of reasons, depending on the age of the child. In line with the idea that the purpose of guilt is to motivate us to detect and heal relationships that we have harmed, parenting provides fertile ground for this emotion to emerge. Just as young children form attachment relationships with their parents, parents develop attachments to their children that start earlier and are at least as intense. Before birth, the mother has a relationship with her unborn child unlike any other. As Shannon described it to me, "It was when I started to feel her move that I felt like this is a little human alive inside of me. I immediately felt love and protective toward her. I started to sit in the rocking chair we had placed in her nursery and sing her the songs that my father had sung to me. I wanted her to recognize them after she was born, so that she would have something familiar between us."

Fathers and adoptive parents are not given the same physical experience with their unborn child as are birth mothers, but there is still plenty of opportunity to fall in love. I remember the first ultrasound, when our daughter's face came into view. The grainy black and white image resembled a skull, but it was *my daughter's* skull. From that moment, she was a real person to me too, and the roots of love could take hold in me as well.

Once the baby is born, parental love explodes. Many new parents describe the experience of birth as love at first sight. Even those mothers who have particularly difficult birthing experiences and are too physically drained or in pain to fully take in the experience of seeing their newborn for the first time report falling in love within hours or days.[*]

And let's be clear that going through pregnancy and childbirth is not necessary to fall in love at first sight with your child. One adoptive parent describes her experience of meeting her adoptive child for the

---

[*] The naturalness of falling in love with your newborn is why postpartum depression can be so harrowing. For those mothers who, for whatever reason, do not immediately fall in love, the negative emotional fallout can be very serious.

first time: "I actually knew I'd love him even before I met him, but seeing him made it all real. I've never felt so protective; I just knew he needed us and we needed him."[2]

Even if they come into the world a bit wrinkled and messy, babies, like all young animals, are designed to be cute. Their cuteness draws adults to them and seduces those adults to look after them. This attribute is important because human babies are comprehensively unable to look after themselves. They are utterly dependent on others, most notably their parents. Parents have almost complete responsibility for the care of their children from birth. This responsibility lasts for years, and although it declines over childhood, parents in Western cultures in particular retain significant responsibility for their children's well-being late into adolescence and even early adulthood.

Together, these two features of parenting—the intense parental love for the child and the long-lived dependence of the child on the parent—create a situation uniquely primed for guilt. With the responsibility of parenting comes multiple possibilities for causing harm, either directly or through negligence. Of course, many of these possibilities are imaginary or of minimal risk, but that doesn't reduce their potency. Thanks to prenatal advice, mothers, even prior to birth, may feel guilty about enjoying a morning coffee or a glass of wine at night. For the next two decades, parents—again, particularly in Western cultures—worry about the health and well-being of their child.

Are they feeding them the right foods? Too much? Too little?

Are they letting their child have too much screen time for optimal cognitive development?[3]

Are they providing the right kind or level of discipline so that their child will grow up to be a good and well-adjusted person?

The dependence of the child on the parent could absorb all their time and energy, but parents inevitably have other concerns. They have other relationships that need to be nurtured—with partners, other children, or perhaps aging parents, who also deserve their attention. They must continue to work to be able to afford the care that their child needs and deserves. They have their own interests and motivations, which also must be nurtured (parents may crave "me time," in which they get to do those things they so enjoyed before parenthood came along). These other commitments inevitably take away attention from their child, and so parenting becomes a constant challenge to balance competing demands.

While parents may need to ration their time and energy toward different activities in addition to childcare, young children almost always want more from their parents than their parents can give them. There is even a term in evolutionary biology for this: "parent-offspring conflict." First coined nearly fifty years ago by biologist Robert Trivers, whom we met in Chapter 2, it is widespread in animals that show intensive parental care, including birds and mammals, especially.[4] In some birds, parents spend all their time foraging for food for their voracious chicks, but even this is sometimes not enough. Raptor chicks are known to try to kill their siblings in the nest to get more of the food their parents provide.[5] In mammals, as we will see a bit later in this chapter, weaning is often a battleground for parent-offspring conflict, where the offspring demands access to the breast beyond the time that the mother wishes to provide it.

The general point is that young children will be as pushy as they can be to get their parents to focus on their needs. As a result, parents often have to say no to their children's demands. Even if you know that saying no to your child is for their own good, and yours, it doesn't mean that it won't pull on your heartstrings. And children's persistence can be frustrating and annoying, so parents may finally respond with angry rebuttals and even physical aggression, such as spanking. This conflict is often seen in an extreme form with the onset of the "terrible twos"—that phase in early development when toddlers start to show strong will and defiance, often leading to tantrums when they do not get what they want.

Mackenzie's first terrible twos meltdown came during an academic conference that Shannon and I were attending in Virginia Beach in 2001. Mackenzie wanted to get into the swimming pool with her shoes on, and when we wouldn't let her, she collapsed on the ground in protest and would not move. Shannon had to pick her up and carry her screaming through the hotel, into the elevator, and up to our room, where she pounded on the door and screamed to get out. All Shannon could think was *What have I done? I have broken my child!* With all these complex concerns, it is no surprise that parents often experience guilt in connection with parenting.

In addition to the genuine responsibilities thrust upon all parents by the dependence of their children, mothers in particular also have to contend with a layer of societal expectations, sometimes known as the "motherhood myth," or what *Time* magazine called, a little more extravagantly, the "Goddess Myth" in 2017.[6] This myth is the idealized concept of the good mother as the person with primary responsibility for the health, well-being, and development of her child, irrespective of the roles that the father or others may play. In the motherhood myth, mothers are cast as essential to the care and development of the child; their mothering powers come perfectly naturally, and they are completely fulfilled in their roles as mothers. Mothers who feel like they are not living up to this ideal, no matter how unrealistic, often report feeling guilt and shame.

I want to emphasize that the motherhood myth really is a myth. While it is perfectly natural for mothers to be caregivers for their children, the idea that it is natural to be a perfect mother is misleading and harmful. Like any role we take on, there is always a huge amount of learning "on the job" for parents. That's why there are so many books, magazines, and websites devoted to helping parents. Furthermore, the idea that mothers should be able to do it by themselves is simply wrong. Within the animal world, humans are what are known as "cooperative breeders," which means that childcare is shared among multiple helpers in addition to the mother.[7] Cooperative breeding is relatively rare in animals, but in every known human society, while mothers generally do invest more time and energy than anyone else in looking after their own children, this maternal investment is augmented by support from others, including fathers, grandparents, older siblings of the child, other relatives (most often female), and unrelated supporters, who may or may not be compensated for providing childcare. The need for all this support gives genuine substance to the African proverb "It takes a village to raise a child." The idea that mothers should be able to do it all alone (and perfectly to boot!) is an unfortunate product of the Western form of social organization known as the nuclear family, which locates child-rearing within the narrow confines of an isolated two-parent family.

With this background, let's look at some of the most common circumstances leading to guilt in parents. So far in this book, I have been making a strong argument that guilt is mostly a good thing. It alerts us to when there may be damage to our relationships and motivates us to try to repair the damage. And this is definitely true for the guilt that parents feel. But we will see also that the conditions that elicit guilt in parents—most obviously the intense love for the child, the desire for them to develop into the best versions of themselves, and the dependence of the child on the parent—can mean that guilt is too easy to come by and can sometimes be counterproductive. Sometimes, the parent will feel guilty for what they need to do, even though it is the right course of action for the health of the child and of the parent-child relationship.

Guilt in Relation to Breastfeeding

Breastfeeding serves at least two important roles in the development of the relationship between mother and newborn. First, of course, breastfeeding is nature's way for mothers to provide nutrition and health care for their infants. There is plenty of good evidence that maternal breast milk provides the best form of nutrition for infants and the greatest health benefits for both infant and mother. For example, infants who are breastfed are at lower risk for developing diabetes and obesity and have better immune system function. Mothers who breastfeed lose pregnancy weight gain faster and appear to be at lower risk for later developing breast and ovarian cancer.[8] This knowledge has led the medical profession over time to implement campaigns of breastfeeding promotion ("Breast is best") to encourage new mothers to opt for breastfeeding over formula. The implicit message is that not breastfeeding will harm the infant, so an effect of such campaigns is to generate guilt in those mothers who are unwilling or unable to breastfeed.

Modern surveys of new mothers show that for mothers who had the intention to breastfeed while they were pregnant, guilt is more prevalent for those who used formula compared to those who were successful in breastfeeding. Mothers who report guilt associated with not breastfeeding often focus on depriving their children of the best nutrition and possibly causing health issues. Unfortunately, such concerns can last a long time. One woman in a study of English new mothers said, "I felt very, very guilty about not being able to breastfeed…every time she has a patch of eczema, I attribute it to the fact that I didn't breastfeed her."[9]

The second role for breastfeeding is in the maintenance of the emotional bond between mother and infant. Unfortunately, this role has been de-emphasized by the medical community that advocates for the physical health benefits of breastfeeding without equal focus on the emotional health benefits of the mother-infant relationship. For Shannon, breastfeeding was a kind of halfway house between the complete protection she provided prior to birth and the inevitable transition of her child into a fully independent person. The guilt she felt was in not being able to deliver on the emotional as well as nutritional benefits during that transition.

Prior to birth, the connection between mother and child is largely bodily; after birth, that bodily connection needs to be replaced by a mostly emotional one. Breastfeeding is an important, although, of course, not essential, way for that transition to occur. There is even a biological basis for this process. Research has shown that the production of oxytocin, the so-called "love hormone," increases during a breastfeeding session, and levels of this hormone remain high when mothers breastfeed exclusively.[10] For some breastfeeding mothers, this approach to feeding their infants also gives them a unique status: no one else can fulfill this role, and so their bond to their infant is special. The guilt that some mothers feel about not breastfeeding is a reaction to the threat to the development of that emotional relationship.

But as Shannon's experience showed, persevering with trying to breastfeed can also be counterproductive when it doesn't work well. For Shannon and Mackenzie, breastfeeding became more and more aversive for both of them as it failed to settle into a natural rhythm. Those moments that should have been filled with joy and comfort were becoming painful and fraught. The switch to formula allowed them to recover swiftly. Although the guilt over the breastfeeding failure persisted, the rebound in the quality of their emotional connection was worth it. Shannon remembers that when she gave up breastfeeding and turned to formula, the serenity of the feeding experience was a revelation. "We were able to sit together calmly in the rocking chair. I would rock and sing while she ate. I wasn't torturing her or me anymore, and that's when I felt that our bonding really began."

I should note that new mothers' breastfeeding experiences are by no means uniform. Even for those mothers who succeed in breastfeeding, the demands on their time and body can feel oppressive. Certainly, breastfeeding is an invasion of mothers' autonomy to live their lives as they had previously. They may express resentment at having to give over their bodies and time to the demands of their new infant. Some mothers have difficulty reconciling the roles of mother and sexual partner, given the dual role of breasts in women's lived experience, and may even feel guilt in connection to the impact of their breastfeeding on their relationship with their partners. These feelings of frustration about meeting their own personal needs may be quickly followed by guilt about resenting their child's needs and not living up to the impossible ideal of the perfect mother.

At the other end of the breastfeeding journey, weaning presents a classic case of parent-offspring conflict. In many mammals, the mother is motivated to wean her offspring as early as possible so she can breed again, while her offspring are motivated to remain breastfeeding as long as possible to focus the mother's attention on them. The human case is a bit more complicated, and some children self-wean even without encouragement. Nevertheless, weaning is often an event that causes considerable conflict between mothers and children.

There is not much scientific research on the extent to which mothers feel guilt in relation to weaning, but even a superficial search of the internet reveals its prevalence. Almost every parenting website that discusses weaning references the guilt that mothers feel, particularly when the weaning is mother-led. It's also clear that this guilt that mothers feel about weaning is not in reaction to medical advice, which is typically limited to breastfeeding for the first six to nine months. Mothers report guilt when they wean their children at any age. The reason, of course, is that mother-led weaning is usually met with child resistance, sadness, and even anger. No mother wants to cause this distress to their child, especially when it is so tied to such a unique and emotionally significant aspect of their relationship with their child.

Guilt in Work-Family Conflict

In many traditional societies, parental leave is nonexistent. Mothers return to their labor as soon as they are physically able, and if they can, they bring their infants strapped to their bodies so there is no separation. For many working parents in Western industrialized societies, the return to work more often entails a separation from their new child, and this separation makes for a challenging time. Managing the demands of work and parenting is a potent source of guilt.

Shannon recalled her experience of this conflict vividly to me:

> I remember when I had the offer to go back to take up a teaching position after being home with Mackenzie for eighteen months. I wasn't really ready to go back to teaching, but I was feeling guilty about not contributing to the family income, and I knew it had to happen sometime, so I agreed to take the position. That first day when we dropped her off at the sitter's was traumatic for me. I cried so hard when we left, and I couldn't do it again, so you remember you had to do it from then on. Over the next few days and weeks, I would go to school and feel guilty that I was leaving *my* child with a sitter to go teach other people's children. But I also felt the pressure to be a good teacher, and I would bring work home with me. I would sometimes feel that Mackenzie was being too demanding when I was at home, so I would get cross with her and feel guilty about that. Then, I would feel I wasn't spending enough quality time with Mackenzie. So, after a while, I felt guilty that I wasn't being a good mom or a good teacher.*

Shannon's story illustrates what is known as "work-family conflict." Work-family conflict is the experience that parents have about the competing demands of their home life and their family life. This conflict is stressful, and guilt is a common part of the experience. Like Shannon, parents often feel the conflict in both directions: family demands can interfere with work, and work demands can interfere with parenting.

---

* Of course, this kind of reaction to returning to work is not universal. A close friend of ours who has a daughter the same age as ours admitted to quite the opposite reaction. She recalled that as her maternity leave was coming to an end and she prepared to return to work, "I couldn't wait; I felt I was so limited staying at home, and I just wanted to get back out there!"

University of California at Irvine professor Jessica Borelli and her colleagues developed the Work Interfering with Family Guilt Scale to assess how mothers and fathers feel about how their work impacts their parenting.[11] The scale is shown below. If you are, or have been, a working mother or father, you can try it for yourself.

Answer each of the questions on a scale of 1 to 5 according to how often you felt this way. Use the key at the bottom of the table. You may notice that some questions are framed to address concerns about work impacting family, and others are framed to explore pride in work. Questions 2, 3, 6, and 9 directly assess how often you feel that your work interferes with your family responsibilities. For these questions, enter your score directly in the final column. Questions 1, 4, 5, 7, and 8 assess your positive feelings about work and how it relates to family life. For these questions, subtract your score from 6 and enter it in the final column. Then add up your total score.

In studies using this scale, the average score is in the mid-20s, which indicates some, but not excessive, guilt. Feeling some guilt is perfectly normal. But if you scored in the mid-30s or higher, you are probably suffering too much from guilt and may need to find a way to reconcile your work and family responsibilities.

How often do you…	Rating*
Feel proud of your role as a worker?	
Feel like you really should be at home when you're away at work?	
Feel guilty about being away from your child when you work longer hours than usual?	
Feel like you should be working when you are at home?	

Feel like working makes you a better parent? ☐

Worry about the impact of your work on your child? ☐

Feel like you contribute to your family through your work? ☐

Feel like your work has a positive impact on your child? ☐

Feel like your decision to work was selfish? ☐

TOTAL ☐

*1 = Never   2 = Rarely   3 = Sometimes   4 = Often   5 = Always

When I learned about this questionnaire and answered it myself, I scored 15, a very low score on work interfering with family guilt (the minimum possible score is 9 and the maximum is 45). If anything, my perennial guilt about not working hard enough led me to feel more guilty about not spending enough time on work! And, despite the changing nature of gender roles in work and parenting, it is still the case that, as the primary caregivers for young children, mothers feel rather more stress and guilt than fathers in relation to the conflict between work and family life. For example, Jessica Borelli and her colleagues gave their Work Interfering with Family Guilt Scale to over a thousand American parents of children between one and three years after they had returned to work. They found that, on average, mothers reported higher scores than fathers did, and this difference was particularly strong for those who worked longer hours outside the home.[12] Similar studies of mothers and fathers in various countries, including the Netherlands and Turkey, have been consistent in showing that mothers are more likely to feel guilty about the impact of the demands of work on their family responsibilities than are fathers.[13] This difference between mothers and fathers seems to be widespread across all cultures whether or not society has traditional gender role expectations with respect to parenting.

This is not to say that fathers do not experience any guilt from work interfering with family; they do, but measurably less so than mothers. Studies of fathers' experience of guilt in relation to work-family conflict suggest that fathers who hold more egalitarian views about the relative roles of mothers and fathers in child-care experience more guilt over their work responsibilities interfering with family than fathers who hold more traditional views. In contrast, more traditional fathers, who see their role as the provider for the family, are more likely to experience guilt when their family responsibilities interfere with their work.[14]

Why do mothers feel more guilt than fathers when work interferes with parenting responsibilities? Researchers often point to societal expectations for mothers. As we have seen in the context of breastfeeding, according to the motherhood myth, the mother is seen as particularly important for the well-being and development of their child. When the demands of work interfere with parenting, mothers may perceive their situations as a failure to live up to this myth of the idealized mother, and, as a result, they feel guilt. As with breastfeeding, the idea here is that guilt arises from the violation of a societal norm.

I think it is important also to recognize that mothers have typically developed more intense relationships with their children because of their greater involvement in early care. As we saw in Chapter 3, the first attachment relationship occurs between an infant and the person who provided the most child-care in early infancy, and this is most commonly the mother. This means that when work interferes with parenting, mothers are more sensitive to the impact of their work demands on their relationships with their children.

In this context, it is interesting to reflect on the impact that progressive approaches to parental leave have had on work-family conflict. Many Western nations now have paid parental leave provisions of twelve months or more. In Canada, for example, parents can take a year of leave with government benefits. The bulk of this leave is "parental," meaning that either parent can take the leave benefit, but in practice, it is much more common, at least in heterosexual couples, for the mother to stay home with the child for most of the leave provision. This situation has two connected consequences. On the one hand, it means mothers spend far more time with their infants during the first year of life than do fathers, and consequentially, their relationship is that much stronger. On the other hand, women experience more longer-term negative impact on their career advancement as well as financial status as a result. Opportunities for career advancement are more likely to pass by those (women or men) who opt to take time out to care for children. Furthermore, as Claudia Goldin of Harvard University showed in her 2023 Nobel Prize–winning research in economics, the wage gap between men and women doing the same job grew after the birth of a first child.[15] It is no real surprise, then, that women experience more work-family conflict.

So what are the consequences of the guilt that results from work-family conflict? There are three kinds of consequences. First, guilt could lead parents to limit, or even terminate, their work, assuming they have the financial flexibility to do so. That way, the source of the work interference on parenting would be lessened, thereby alleviating guilt. It is a fact that women are more likely than men to be lost from the workforce after having children. Although in most cases, we cannot know to what extent guilt plays a role, studies of working parents have shown that many of them do regularly think about ways they might reduce their work commitments. Lianne Aarntzen of Utrecht University in the Netherlands and her colleagues asked a group of working mothers to fill out a diary every day for a week that recorded their guilt, their thoughts about reducing work commitments, and their overall happiness. She found that mothers who reported high levels of guilt also regularly reported thinking of ways to reduce their work commitments.[16]

Second, because the guilt is experienced as a negative emotional state, one might imagine that there would be consequences for parents' overall emotional well-being. In her study of guilt in working mothers, Aarntzen found that mothers who reported more guilt also reported more overall unhappiness in relation to their work-family conflict. There is some indication that for many working mothers, it is the guilt in relation to their perceived failure to meet the demands of the motherhood myth that contributes to an overall deterioration in emotional well-being.

The third consequence is that if guilt results from concerns about the way work is impacting their family relationships, then you could imagine that parents might change the way they parent their children. And, indeed, research has shown that guilt does affect parenting approaches.

Guilt and Parenting Style

An important dimension when considering parenting is not just whether or not parents try to control their children's behavior, but *how much* control they try to exert over their children's behavior. This dimension can be considered to range from permissive to controlling. Permissive parenting is a relatively hands-off approach. Parents provide less guidance to their children overall and are more likely to give in to children's demands. In contrast, controlling parenting is when parents give children little freedom and try to keep their children on a tight leash so that they will conform to what the parents want them to do.[17] As I'm sure you can imagine, neither extremely permissive nor extremely controlling parenting is ideal. It is generally believed that a moderate degree of guidance, while allowing children to develop a healthy degree of autonomy, is best.

Research that has investigated the effect of parental guilt on parenting has pointed to two possible impacts. First, in line with the idea that parental guilt arises because of feeling that they are neglecting or damaging their relationship with their children, parents may attempt to repair the relationship by overindulging their children, giving in to them, and becoming more permissive. In their study of work impacting family guilt, Jessica Borelli and her colleagues found that parents who reported higher levels of guilt were more likely to suggest permissive responses to hypothetical situations where their child was upset, such as offering candy.[18]

Parental guilt is not only related to how indulgent parents are; it can also have an impact on how controlling parents are, although in this case, the connection is a bit more complicated. Research has reliably shown that parents who feel that their personal or professional interests have been frustrated by the amount of time and energy that they must devote to parenting often respond by increasing the amount of control they exert over their children.[19] Ortal Slobodin and her colleagues at Ben-Gurion University found that parental guilt moderated this effect. This means that parents who felt guilty about the way they were parenting were less likely to increase their control in reaction to feeling that their other interests were being frustrated. So here, perhaps unsurprisingly, guilt appears to reduce the extent to which parents show a controlling approach to parenting their children when they are frustrated that they have less time for their other activities.[20]

In addition to how parents go about managing their children's behavior, one can also look at the kinds of activities that parents do with their children. A simple categorization is to think of activities as educational (for example, reading), recreational (for example, playing), and passive (which these days mostly means "screen time," such as watching TV together). Not surprisingly, competing demands on parents' time can impact the ability of parents to engage in these activities with their children, and this interference often leads to guilt. So, how does this guilt affect how parents engage with their children? In a study of several hundred parents, Eunae Cho and Tammy Allen of the University of South Florida found that parents who reported competing work demands engaged with their children less across all types of interaction.[21] However, parents who reported more guilt were less likely to let competing work demands interfere with their educational and recreational parenting activities. What this means is that feeling guilt can help parents maintain their active engagement with their children.

Guilt and Divorce

Let's finish this tour of circumstances leading to parents' guilt in relation to their children with perhaps the most extreme situation: the breakdown in the parents' relationship ending in divorce. It used to be the case that divorce required the identification of a guilty or an at-fault party. That more legalistic approach no longer applies in most Western societies, which have adopted a no-fault approach to divorce. Nevertheless, divorce can generate a painful mixture of guilty feelings because of the many relationships that may be negatively impacted, including with the ex-spouse, family members, in-laws, and perhaps wider social relations within social groups and institutions, such as churches. But divorce is particularly hard on children. Inevitably, the changes in custody after divorce will cause some disruption to the relationships that have been established between parents and their children. Many studies have shown that children experience a decline in emotional well-being after their parents' divorce (at least in the short term).[22] The typical result for any parent who cares about their child is feeling guilt for being the cause of the emotional impact on their child and the relationship disruption. Parents may also feel guilt from the failure to meet society's expectations about maintaining an intact two-parent family unit, which is taken to be the best model for raising children.

A large-scale study of parents in the Netherlands explored these ideas by asking divorced and still-married parents to report on their feelings of guilt in relation to their oldest child.[23] The parents also reported on the quality of their relationship with their children by rating statements such as "I am very fond of my child" and "I am often angry with my child." Finally, the parents were asked a series of questions to get at their endorsement of traditional societal attitudes to marriage, such as whether parents should be married to have children. The results showed that parents who were divorced were more than twice as likely to report guilt in connection with their children than parents who were still married. There was no difference between mothers and fathers in this regard; both reported much more guilt if they were divorced. When the researchers looked at how the quality of the parents' relationship with their children affected guilt, they found that the difference in guilt between married and divorced parents was greater for those parents who enjoyed more *positive* relationships with their children. In other words, the stronger the parent-child relationship, the more divorced parents felt guilt compared to married parents. Divorce clearly provokes guilt in parents toward their children, and the closer the parents feel toward their children, the more guilty divorced parents feel. Parents who held more traditional ideas about the importance of marriage for child-rearing also reported more guilt than those with more liberal views, so there also seemed to be a contribution to guilt of contravening societal norms.

When she heard I was writing this book, a friend of mine, Emily, shared with me her feelings as her marriage with her two children's father was unraveling nearly twenty years ago. While she had no regrets about her decision to separate from her husband—the marriage had broken down irretrievably—the guilt Emily experienced about the impact of the family breakdown on her children, who were ten and thirteen at the time, was severe. The children were clearly hurting. One of them told her, "My life was perfect and happy and everything was great until you and Daddy gave me the news that you weren't going to live together anymore, and my world fell apart." Emily described hearing that as a punch to the gut. The other refused to stay at their mother's new home for many months and eventually had to be bribed to do so by the purchase of a bearded dragon. Knowing that she had instigated their pain felt awful, and there was no immediate relief. She couldn't apologize to her children for leaving their father, and they certainly were not in a position to forgive her. Furthermore, as the one who had initiated the separation, Emily was too easily cast as the home-breaker by her extended family and mutual friends. She was the one who had failed to live up to the image of, as she described it, "the perfect wife, perfect mother, in a perfect marriage." So, inevitably, her guilt in connection to her children was compounded by guilt about harming the whole network of family relationships. But at the same time, Emily had no doubts that the decision to separate was the right one. She told me that the first night she stayed in her new home, she slept better than she had in years. Soon, she was able to find herself again and, most importantly, find a way to parent that was right for her and for her children. Now, almost twenty years after her divorce, Emily has a wonderful relationship with her adult children, and she has become the center of family life—her home is the place where all of the extended family come together for celebrations.

How, then, should parents who have decided to divorce go about managing their guilt in relation to the children? It is important to remember that although children will almost certainly be hurt emotionally when their parents separate, that does not mean that staying together is better for the children. Conflict in the marriage is also harmful for children. The comparison may seem superficial, but Emily's story reminded me of Shannon's fight with Mackenzie over breastfeeding. If a relationship with one's children is suffering from doing things the "right" way, it is surely better to switch and do it "your" way. The guilt may still linger, but the relationship can get stronger, and that, as we have seen, is the real value of guilt. Then, one can look back, empathize with the self that had to cause the initial pain, and forgive that self for what they had to do.

Pet Parent Guilt

The Covid-19 pandemic, during which time many people were largely confined at home, and the subsequent return to the workplace have brought to light a different manifestation of parental guilt. During the height of the pandemic, many pet parents* spent much more time with their pets and subsequently experienced guilt about leaving their pets when they had to return to the workplace. This reaction should not be a surprise. Pet-parent relationships have some similarities to child-parent relationships. In particular, there is a strong and mutually affectionate connection between the parent and pet, with the parent having almost complete responsibility for the well-being of the highly dependent pet. As with children, the ingredients are there for parental guilt to arise.

I know the feeling! We got our first dog—Scamper, a Yorkshire terrier—thirteen years ago. As the default family dog walker, I would take him out for a walk every evening. But then, eight years later, we got another: Bear, a Morkie (Yorkshire-Maltese mix). We had no expectation that caring for two similar dogs of different ages would be much more work, but now neither of them get walked as often as they should. They have completely different walking styles—Bear pulls as he tries to race ahead despite every attempt to train it out of him, while Scamper, now a senior citizen with a reconstructed ACL, is much slower and likes to sniff every blade of grass along the way. These different walking styles inevitably means that they must be walked separately, and I hate to admit that there have been many evenings when the thought of walking one dog and then returning home to take the next one out has meant that neither of them get walked. On those evenings, I can't help feeling guilty that I have neglected their needs.

To get some sense of how widespread guilt is in pet parents, Lori Kogan of Colorado State University and her colleagues conducted a

---

* The use of the word "parent" to describe pet owners is justified. Research has shown that a large majority of pet owners consider their pet to be a member of the family similar in status to human children.

survey of over five hundred American dog owners in the spring of 2022, after the critical period of the pandemic was over and most had returned to the workplace.[24] Using a measure similar to the work-family conflict questionnaire I reviewed earlier, they found that the overall level of guilt in relation to their dogs was very similar to that typically reported in studies of work-family guilt. Almost all pet parents reported some level of guilt, and 30 percent reported that they struggled significantly with guilt. They felt guilty about spending too much time away from their dogs, about not looking after their dogs' needs enough, including walking them as often as they should, and about not being able to provide the best possible health care. So, pet parent guilt is very common. And it is not trivial. In a follow-up study of over six hundred American dog owners, Kogan and her colleagues found that higher levels of dog-related guilt were associated with dog parents tending to avoid social engagements such as evenings out or weekends away.[25] Choosing not to leave a dog for a social event is a choice, but returning to work may not be. Like work-family conflict, pet guilt can be a source of emotional distress. Those who reported more dog-related guilt experienced significantly more stress, including symptoms of depression and anxiety. Kogan and her colleagues suggest that pet parent guilt should be taken seriously as a potential negative contributor to workplace satisfaction and performance.

Parental guilt stems from the intense nature of the parent-child relationship, and it tends to be strongest when the dependence of the child on the parent and the perceived risk of harm are greatest. But, of course, children grow older and become more able to care for themselves. This usually means that, for parents, the risk of contracting parental guilt reduces as their children grow up. That's not to say that parents will gradually run out of guilt as their children mature into adults. One's children will always be one's children, and parents care about them and feel some responsibility for them forever. And guilt can always accompany this feeling of a responsibility of care. But as children become more capable, the parent's responsibility of caring decreases and with it the pervasiveness of the guilt.

So, how should parents deal with their guilt in relation to their children? Let's remember first that given the strength of the parent-child bond and the need for parents to provide for, control, and sometimes discipline their children, it is almost inevitable that parents will feel guilt from time to time. Parents can't help but empathize with their children, and they regularly feel anxious about their children's well-being. Children often resist their parents' control, and so conflict regularly arises. In those moments, parents may fear that their children's love for them is at risk. So, the emotional ingredients for guilt—empathy and anxiety—are omnipresent. Finally, there is no perfect user manual for how to parent, and so it is easy for parents to question their parenting decisions and feel like they are making mistakes. These circumstances make guilt in relation to their children an almost universal experience for parents, and especially mothers.

Parenting guilt arises in all kinds of circumstances. But how much of this guilt is really warranted? Remember that the purpose of guilt is to heal potentially damaged relationships, and healing occurs through the acceptance of wrongdoing, apology, and forgiveness by the other. This approach to guilt provides a useful guide to when parenting guilt should be listened to and when it can be ignored and let go. Parents may ask themselves whether they need to apologize to their child for what they did and commit to not doing it again. In some cases, the answer is obvious. Shannon does not need to apologize to Mackenzie for not breastfeeding her. The development of their relationship was being hampered by their breastfeeding troubles, and it improved immediately after the bottle was introduced. Although Shannon felt guilt at the time, it was not useful and eventually dissipated.

In other cases, there is more ambiguity. Imagine a parent yelling at a child for not following a request to help clean up after dinner (again). The child becomes sullen and withdrawn, and the parent feels guilty for damaging the health of the relationship. The parent needs to ask themselves what their responsibility for the harm to the relationship is. Here, the parenting directive is reasonable even if the way it was delivered, while understandable, is not. Perhaps an apology is warranted for the angry delivery but not for its content. The parent could apologize for yelling but explain why they got so frustrated and why the directive is important. In this case, the parent stays firm in their parenting directive but moves from an assertion of power to an inductive mode of parenting, confirming that they care about the child and their relationship even if certain rules still must apply.

So, if you are a parent who is stricken by parental guilt, ask yourself: *Do I need my child to forgive me for how I acted?* If you answer no, then let go of the guilt—it is misplaced.

Chapter Seven

Guilt and Adult Children

"It happened again!" Shannon said, turning to look at me as I walked out of my home office to take a break from working on the manuscript for this book. She had just gotten off the phone with her ninety-year-old mother, who lives in an independent living retirement community close to our house. I could see the frustration in the set of Shannon's face and a hint of sadness in her eyes.

"What happened?"

"She just told me again how Sheila's daughter took her out for ice cream yesterday."

"Did *she* want to go out for ice cream?"

"I didn't ask. I just said, 'Well, Sheila has three daughters, who all live close by.' Why did I need to say that? I know she didn't tell me just to make me feel bad, so why do I react like that?" She slumped onto the couch and stared out of the bay window.

"You were frustrated. It's not like you don't do so much for her already."

"I know, but I feel so guilty when she says those things."

I sat down next to her on the couch and gave her a hug. After a minute or two, Shannon was up and walking over to the phone again. She had to call the drugstore to make sure that her mother's prescriptions had been filled and were ready for pickup.

These days, this kind of experience is a regular occurrence for Shannon in her everyday interactions with her mother. And to be clear, an offhand comment from her mother isn't required to stimulate the guilt. Shannon is constantly aware of whether she is doing enough for her mother. She is the only one of her immediate family living close by. Her father passed away some years ago, and Shannon has been her mother's close companion ever since. Her mother gave up driving a few years ago, limiting her independence, and while she is still lively enough in one-on-one conversation, she has begun to get confused easily. Shannon now schedules and attends every medical appointment with her, takes her shopping, manages her finances, and troubleshoots when something goes wrong with her iPad or TV. Conservatively, the time commitment is equivalent to at least a half-time job—not that she thinks of it that way.

Shannon is completing the journey of her mother-daughter relationship from dependent child through equal adult to adult carer for her aging parent. As a child, Shannon idolized her glamorous and accomplished mother—one of the first women to host a news program on Canadian television in the 1950s. In her late teens, after dropping out of her first university degree, Shannon moved away from her parents to establish her own identity and career. She then returned to her hometown in her thirties to live close to her parents, and as adults, she and her mother spent many years as close confidantes and even best friends. Now, she has added the role of caregiver that her mother needs as her health, mobility, and cognitive acuity decline.

Through all the transitions in the lifelong history of parent-child relationships, guilt has a part to play. We have already seen how guilt appears in the lives of young children and their parents. In Chapter 3, we saw that children need to ensure that they are cared for by their parents, and so they experience guilt when they fear that they have done something to threaten their parents' love for them. Their guilt keeps them inclined to conform to their parents' demands, which become internalized as conscience and a source of guilt throughout life. In the previous chapter, we saw how, for their part, parents are carers who want to do the best for their developing children, and they experience guilt when they are concerned that they have in some way not done enough or perhaps harmed their child. The guilt keeps them focused on providing as much high-quality care as possible. In the final phase of the child-parent relationship, these two forms of guilt may merge as the adult child feels both the guilt of the child and the guilt of the carer simultaneously. Shannon feels guilt when she thinks she has fallen short of what her mother expects of her, and, at the same time, she feels guilt when she senses that she has not provided the care her mother needs.*

In between these two bookends of the life course of the child-parent relationship, there is the period that can help to make or break how the relationship is managed in the long term: how parents and their children manage their relationship as the maturing children seek their independence from the family of origin. And, once again, we will see that guilt has an important role to play. In this chapter, we will first look at the role of guilt in managing the relationship between parents and their children as the latter develop into independent adults. Then, we will turn our attention to how guilt plays into the relationships between aging adults and their family caregivers.

Guilt in Emerging Adults

I have said very little in this book so far about the period of adolescence or its immediate developmental neighbor, emerging adulthood.[1] I do not mean to imply that this period is free of guilt for either parents or their children. In fact, it is quite the opposite. Adolescence and emerging adulthood is a time when the relationship between child and parent can become genuinely strained—and sometimes broken at least temporarily—as adult children seek to develop an identity outside of the structure of the family. Children may make choices that parents do not approve of. And parents may attempt to exert control over their children that is resisted. Along with this tension in the relationship can come guilt on both sides. Parents may feel guilt for the parenting decisions that they worry may have contributed to the tension. For their part, adolescents and young adults may resent parental control but feel guilt for not following their parents' wishes.

---

* Shannon knows that the responsibility for caring she feels toward her mother and the guilt that accompanies that responsibility is only a mild case of what many carers of aging loved ones feel. She was there twenty years ago to assist her mother, who was the primary caregiver for her father as he rapidly deteriorated with early onset Alzheimer's in his late sixties. After he became a risk to himself and Shannon's mother while living at home, they had to make the difficult decision to put him in respite care at a residential long-term care facility, and he died there shortly after.

Tension in the parent-child relationship arises because as children pass through adolescence and develop into adults, the nature of their relationship changes. Research on how adult children and their parents view their relationship has reliably shown that parents are more invested in the relationship than their adult children are. And adult children generally view their relationships with their parents less positively than their parents do.[2] Parents retain an interest in providing support where they can for their maturing children, particularly when they are starting out as adults. Their focus in their relationship with their children is to ensure that their children thrive and continue to develop in the way they feel is best. They take an interest in the success, both career and familial, of their children, and are eager to play a role in ensuring that success. Whether success means a certain type of career or lifestyle or family, most parents want their children to be all that they can be. Parents, especially as they age beyond their own careers, are also more concerned with the continuity between the generations, and may be especially keen on supporting their children's own families.

Beginning in adolescence, children's relationship interests and motivations take on a different focus. Of course, they still love their parents. Their relationships with their parents remain some of the most important ones for adult children across cultures.[3] But while they may continue to seek and receive security from their parents, adolescents start to look outwards, away from their family of origin. As adults, children are primarily focused on achieving their own goals, whether for career or family. Adult children explore and develop new significant relationships outside the family, with friends, with romantic partners, with work colleagues. In time, their most significant relationships will likely become their romantic partners and their own children, if they have them. Inevitably, their focus will shift predominantly to these relationships and away from their own parents.

So, it is not surprising that parents and their adult children are invested in their mutual relationships to differing degrees. You might say that parents and adult children are working toward the same general goals—the interests of the adult children—but they may not agree on exactly what those goals should be or on how to achieve them.[4] And this, of course, is where tension can arise in the relationship.

As their children mature into adults, parents are presented with a choice: should they continue to exert a degree of control over their adult children as they did when their children were young, or should they relinquish control and let their children make their own choices in life. I think we can all agree that, in principle, when teaching one's child to drive, there comes a time when the parent must take their hands off the steering wheel. But we also recognize that this is not always so easy to do, especially when it might appear that the child is heading toward the ditch! Relinquishing control is made all the more difficult when adult children are reluctant to fully commit to independence, perhaps living at home in their parents' basement or regularly asking for financial support.

In addition to having an opinion on how their children should lead their lives, parents may have a view on their children's responsibility to them, sometimes called "filial obligation."[5] Parents may believe that their children, even as adults, have a duty to respect them, follow their wishes, and perhaps transition into caring more for them as they age. They may attempt to exert control over their adult children with respect to such obligations. There are reliable cultural and individual differences in the extent to which filial obligation is expected by parents. In particular, filial obligation is assumed to a much greater degree in collectivist cultures compared to individualist ones.[6] And, at least in Western cultures, it appears that parents who show an anxious attachment style are more likely to believe that their children have an obligation to provide care for them when necessary.[7]

Parental control is the single most significant source of tension or conflict in the parent–adult child relationship. And as anyone who has parented (or indeed been) an adolescent will understand, this tension comes in like a relationship wrecking ball in the years between childhood and adulthood.

Adolescents are highly sensitive to being controlled by their parents. Although they may still be content to enjoy the security of what the family context provides, they want the freedom to explore life experiences away from the confines of the family. One (perhaps *the*) important psychological task of this period of life is to develop an identity that is personal and feels unique and authentic. This task will take some years to complete, but most adolescents and emerging adults want to accomplish it without too much parental intervention. Once the task is completed, adult children may begin to develop their relationship with their parents on a new footing.

For parents, this period of their children's development presents a difficult challenge. The task of parenting is not yet complete, but how much control over their children's behavior is appropriate and how much coercion should be applied? Researchers interested in this question have explored the kinds of control that parents offer their adolescent children and how well these methods sit with their offspring.

One innovative approach was carried out by Brian Barber and his colleagues working in collaboration with the World Health Organization.[8] They asked adolescents in different cultures in Costa Rica, Thailand, and South Africa to identify the kinds of things that their parents did or said that made them feel disrespected as individuals. There was considerable agreement from adolescents in the different cultures, suggesting that, across the world, adolescents have similar concerns about how their parents attempt to control them. These concerns include being ridiculed and embarrassed in front of others, having unrealistic expectations for them, and being made to feel guilty about things they had done. These parental control tactics appear to be the most poisonous with respect to the quality of the parent-adolescent relationship. They tend to make adolescents less respectful of their parents' wishes and less interested in sharing information about their lives. They also tend to be associated with psychological problems in adolescence, such as signs of depression.[9]

In a study of American adolescents, Wendy Rote and Judith Smetana examined how parental guilt induction in particular can affect adolescent feelings.[10] They compared how adolescents viewed guilt induction in connection to both moral issues and personal choices, and how they felt about guilt induction where the parent tried to make the adolescent feel guilty in relation to the person who had been hurt versus in relation to the parent themselves. Overall, adolescents had little problem with guilt induction about moral issues or when the focus was on someone who had been harmed: "You know you hurt Claire's feelings when you flirted with her boyfriend." But they expressed considerable resentment when parents tried to make them feel guilty about their personal choices by focusing on their own hurt feelings: "It makes me upset when you stay up all night playing video games." Adolescents felt that this kind of parental guilt-induction inhibited their personal autonomy and suggested that their parent was more concerned with themselves than with the well-being of the adolescents. This research on how parents exert control over their adolescent children suggests that the parent–adult child relationship can be damaged by too intrusive an approach to the adult child's independence and autonomy. I should note, however, that cultural differences may exist here also. For example, research has found that guilt-induction in relation to filial obligation was viewed positively by young adults from India but negatively by young adults from the US.[11]

This research on parental control of their adolescent children and particularly the work on guilt induction suggests that a major source of conflict or tension in the parent–adult child relationship is the control tactics that parents use as their children are emerging into adulthood. When young adults perceive their parents to be overly controlling, especially around personal choices, they tend to resist and become resentful. In consequence, as children develop into adults, they will diminish the importance of their relationship with their parents in their everyday lives. They are less likely to share with their parents what is happening in their lives and are more likely to reduce the amount of contact they have with their parents.

In extreme circumstances, the tension between adult children and their parents can lead to estrangement, whereby adult children and their parents have no contact. Estrangements are most often initiated by the child. In a US survey published in 2023, Rin Reczek and their colleagues found that approximately 6 percent of adults have experienced some period of estrangement from their mothers and 26 percent from their fathers.[12] Perhaps fortunately, the majority of those who have been estranged become unestranged in time. Adult children who opt to cut themselves off from their family of origin are often beset by guilt as well as grief. For example, one poster on the Reddit thread *r/Estranged Adult Child* sought feedback from the online community on their experience:

> When do you know if estrangement is best for you? My family tell me I am upsetting my mother for being angry for the abuse she inflicted on me as a child, I am made out to be the bad guy. To the point where I am second guessing it happened. All I can feel is immense guilt at the sadness I am causing my mother even though she is the one who has caused me years of stress and anxiety. How do I shake the guilt and grief?[13]

To my knowledge, there is no formal research on the prevalence of guilt in those who are estranged. However, in line with the idea that guilt serves to motivate relationship repair, it would be interesting to know whether those that feel guilt to a greater extent are more likely to attempt to reconnect in due course than those whose feelings are dominated by other emotions such as anger and grief.

In contrast, when young adults receive guidance and support from their parents that is respectful of their need for independence and autonomy, the relationship can grow in a new direction that embraces the individuality of each. It becomes more of a close friendship, with a long, shared history. Parent and adult child engage in more frequent contact, even if they are not living close to each other. Experiences are shared, advice and support are mutually provided. The strength of the parent-child bond serves them well when the relationship has to shift again in the provision of care, with the child becoming the provider of care for the aging parent.

Guilt in the Care of Seniors

Worldwide, the population is aging.[14] But while people are living longer and healthier lives, time inevitably takes its toll and most elderly people require increasing support in their daily lives. Caring for the elderly becomes most urgent when they lose the ability to care for themselves. The risk of Alzheimer's and related dementias increases significantly after age sixty-five and accelerates after eighty years of age.[15] As cognitive function declines, the responsibilities of caregivers begin to resemble those of parents with young children, except that the need for care increases over time rather than decreases, and with those responsibilities come many opportunities for guilt to emerge.

Inevitably, family members remain the most important source of support and care for the elderly, particularly before physical and mental health has declined to the point where either full-time live-in care or transition to a residential long-term care facility is required. As with childcare, elder care is taken on more commonly by women compared to men.[16] Spouses provide some of this care, but it is the adult children, and most often adult daughters, of the elderly that assume the bulk of the care responsibilities.[17] Women often feel the weight of familial or societal expectations to be the carer for family members in need. Falling short of these demands leads to guilt, and it almost certainly impacts women disproportionately.

Like any experience of guilt, caregiver guilt is a complex emotion. Caregiving for someone with dementia typically incorporates all of the emotional components of guilt. There is the empathic sadness for the other, resulting from their deteriorating health. There is fear over the loss of the relationship as it slips away. And there is often self-blame for not managing to care enough. While spouses of those with dementia experience all these components of guilt, adult children caring for their parents with dementia experience guilt even more intensely. A big part of this difference is that spouses are more likely to have a dedicated focus on their ailing spouse, whereas adult children are often torn between multiple competing relationship responsibilities.

When caregivers for the elderly—both adult children and spouses—are asked about their guilt feelings, they typically report guilt from several sources.[18] The first and perhaps most obvious source of guilt is the feeling of not doing a good enough job of caring for the loved one—that despite one's best efforts, the loved one is suffering, and that suffering continues to grow. In contrast to the experience of parenting, where one sees the rewards of caring in the development and blossoming of one's charges, elder care is often increasingly difficult and unrelentingly demanding work. It is both physically and emotionally draining. And yet, despite these demands, the rewards diminish as the ravages of time continue. Of course, this guilt is misplaced; the caregiver is not responsible for their loved one's suffering, but as we have seen, guilt is not rational. It arises naturally when we see suffering in those we care for and about.

Caregivers, especially adult children, who take on the responsibility of caring for a loved one with dementia are often torn between competing caring responsibilities. More adults these days are stuck in the so-called sandwich generation. Social work professor Dorothy Miller coined this term in 1981 to refer to adults sandwiched between parental responsibilities for their children and caring responsibilities for their aging parents.[19] The sandwich generation has grown over time as many parents delayed having their own children into their thirties or even forties, and so by the time their children are in middle and high school, their own parents may be starting to require significant support and care. A recent study by the Pew Research Center found that almost 25 percent of adults in the US have one or more parents over sixty-five while they are still responsible for their own children. The majority of these adults are between forty and forty-nine years of age.[20] Having active and engaged grandparents around can, of course, be a boon for one's own childcare responsibilities, but as those grandparents age into increasing frailty, adults stuck in the sandwich generation can find themselves with double the caring responsibilities. For those adults living close to their aging parents, these two sets of responsibilities can often collide. And this is before one considers the toll that a double set of caring responsibilities can take on one's feelings of responsibility to one's workplace. At any one time, the carer may feel guilty that they are neglecting one or more of their other responsibilities.

Committing to caring for a loved one doesn't mean that the caregiver will not at times wish that someone else would take it over. If an adult child caregiver has siblings who cannot or will not step up to care for the parent, they may get frustrated that the burden of care has fallen to them rather than their siblings. They may express this frustration and then feel guilty for doing so. Here, the guilt arises from the fact that the carer may blame and be angry or resentful of others that they care about. Paradoxically, caregivers also report feeling guilt when they do take some time for themselves and hand over responsibilities to someone else for a while. Here, the guilt comes from not living up to their own standard of being a good enough carer. When it comes to warding off the demands of caregiving guilt, it seems there is no winning.

Perhaps the most difficult guilt-inducing situation for both spouses and adult children caring for an increasingly frail senior is the decision to move them out of their own home and into a residential long-term care facility. Making this decision brings together many sources of guilt. Unfortunately, it may be seen as an admission of failure—that one cannot be the caregiver that one's loved one needs. If the senior is comfortable with the move, then a significant source of caregiver stress is removed. But, when the senior is upset about the decision and resists the move, caregivers often report feeling guilty that they have abandoned and betrayed their loved one. This experience is particularly common in spouses. As one caregiver spouse put it, "One time I came to visit him…and he just all of a sudden said, 'I'm not here for me, I'm here for you. I'm here because it's easier for you.' I wanted to say, 'I don't know how to take care of you...and the house.' I literally left in tears."[21]

The primary caregivers for seniors often second-guess whether they are making the right decision in moving the senior to a residential long-term care facility. They may worry that their loved one's mental deterioration will be exacerbated by the institutional environment. One spouse mused, "I wonder if his dementia has progressed more because he's not engaged at the facility." But such concerns can often be countered by a transition to a facility that opens up more opportunities for activity and social engagement. A daughter's guilt at making the decision to transition her mother from her home to a residential long-term care facility was relieved when she saw that it "improved her quality of life, social engagement, and, in some ways, has given me peace of mind. She had lived alone for so long, so I think not having a lot of engagement was not good for her."

Caregivers have a unique level of insight into what their loved one needs, but this may not stop others from weighing in with their opinions. Another wife caregiver reported that her husband's dementia had caused him to start acting violently toward her when they were alone. "People say, 'Why did [you move him there] in the first place?' When he's so sweet when they're around, I don't want to say, 'He's not always that way!' I feel bad about saying that. He's been ugly and violent. I'd feel guilty if I said that, like I'm betraying his confidence."

Much of the guilt that arises in the context of elderly caregiving is borne out of empathy for the loved one whose suffering is growing and the feeling of inability to manage it as one would like to be able to do. One might see this as a healthy, compassionate form of guilt even if it may, at times, be misplaced. It can be managed and largely dissipated by a realistic assessment of one's responsibility, an assessment that can be facilitated by a credible external perspective on the situation. Many residential long-term care facilities offer transition counseling to help carers manage the emotional effects of moving their loved one to a facility. Such counseling often targets caregiver guilt and helps provide a necessary external perspective that can alleviate the guilt. After her husband had been settled in a residential long-term care facility, one caregiver wife explained, "I used to feel guilty that I don't have him at home anymore. But it's pretty clear to me, and others that I talk to, that it's not possible to safely take care of him and myself at home. The guilt of that is gone. Not that it won't come back ever."

There is no question that caring for a family member with dementia is stressful. It can be both physically and emotionally draining, and guilt is a common part of the experience. Indeed, the intensity of guilt that caregivers feel contributes significantly to the overall amount of stress they feel.[22] But for some caregivers, the stress of caring can transition into severe emotional distress and even clinical depression.[23] Caregivers may become deeply morose, lacking in energy and in motivation to engage in any regular activities outside of their caregiving role. Why do some carers cope reasonably well with the demands of caregiving whereas others descend into depression? It turns out that guilt plays a role here also. This final form of caregiver guilt is more insidious, and it stems from an undercurrent of resentment toward the loved one and toward the role that the caregiver has taken on.

To try to understand which caregivers experience this guilt, Matthijs Kalmijn of the University of Amsterdam surveyed nearly 2,500 adult children with aging mothers about their feelings toward their parent.[24] The children, the majority of whom were women, averaged forty-three years of age. Kalmijn asked the children to rate both their positive feelings, such as affection, for their mother and their negative feelings, like anger, toward their mother. He also asked them to report how much guilt they felt in connection to their mothers. Not surprisingly, those adult children who felt more positive toward their mothers tended to feel less negative and vice versa. But there was a minority of adult children who reported both strong positive *and* strong negative feelings, and it was these participants who reported the highest levels of guilt in relation to their mothers. Guilt came from being both very close to the parent and being angry at them. Kalmijn's survey suggests that intense guilt can arise when there is ambivalence in the adult child–parent relationship. It turns out that this link between ambivalence and guilt is the most likely reason that some caregivers experience severe mental health deterioration. The caregivers who show indications of depression are the ones who report the most ambivalence in their relationship with their loved one and who also experience the most guilt because of this ambivalence.[25] Furthermore, this depression can persist even after caregiving responsibilities are minimized either because the loved one requires intensive professional care or has passed away. This fact suggests that the negative emotions are not the direct result of feeling that one is not fulfilling one's caregiving responsibilities well enough. There is something deeper at play.

The link between ambivalence, guilt, and depression reminds us that the quality of the relationship between the caregiver and the recipient of care is an important issue for appreciating the emotional landscape of caring for an aging loved one.[26] To understand the dynamics of the caregiver-senior relationship, it helps to think of it in terms of attachment style. Attachments between children and their parents begin in early infancy, and they characterize relationships throughout life, even into old age.[27] The caregiver, whether adult child or spouse, is in an attachment relationship with the senior, and, moreover, the senior is in an attachment relationship with the carer. In this final stage of relationships, the quality of their relationship remains a critical influence on how guilt shows up.

John Bowlby, the originator of attachment theory, considered attachment and caring as complementary aspects of the attachment relationship and argued that the attachment-caring dynamic of our close relationships persists throughout life from "cradle to grave."[28] Attachment is the process by which one person in a close relationship seeks comfort and security from the other. Caring is the way the other person in the relationship provides the sought-for comfort and security. We have looked already at young children's attachment to their parents and at how this attachment can transfer to romantic relationships. In the case of children's attachment to their parents, the parents provide all the caring for the children who seek comfort and security from their parents. In the case of attachment between romantic partners and spouses, the dynamic has a more balanced, symmetrical arrangement: both seek comfort and security from the other and both provide emotional care for the other. But as seniors age into frailty, the attachment dynamic within their relationships shifts. The senior becomes less and less able to be a provider of comfort and security to others and becomes predominantly a recipient of care.

This shift becomes especially pronounced as seniors age into dementia. In the earlier stages of the disease, when the senior is aware of their circumstances, they will experience their cognitive decline with anxiety, and their attachment-related need for security will be transferred onto those loved ones who are available for support—the spouse or adult children. We know that attachments are an important factor for understanding the quality of seniors' relationships because as the disease progresses, and they increasingly lose touch with reality, many seniors acquire the delusion that their own parents, who typically passed away many years earlier, are available to care for them. This delusion is called "parent fixation," and some estimates are that 50 to 60 percent of nursing home residents with dementia believe that one or both parents are available to look after them.[29] They appear to experience the nursing home as a separation from their attachment figure and may ask to go home to their parents. It is as though the senior's attachment system has reverted to its original childlike state.

It's important to understand that just as they had different attachment styles in childhood or in their romantic relationships, the elderly have different attachment styles that will affect how they express and cope with their need for security and care from others.[30] And the way that seniors show their attachment styles can have significant repercussions for those family members who are tasked with their care.[31] Seniors who have a secure attachment style tend to be more content and show more joy in their interactions with loved ones. Their more relaxed demeanor inevitably makes their carers feel more optimistic as well as appreciated in their role. Seniors with anxious attachment styles exhibit more negative emotion, including anxiety and sadness or depression. Some insecurely attached seniors show ambivalent reactions to their carers as they express both neediness for love and attention mixed with anger toward their loved ones. It is easy to see how such emotional reactions from their aging loved ones may create ambivalence and guilt in carers.

The shift in attachment dynamics between a senior and their caregiver, whether spouse or adult child, has important implications for the emotional state of the caregiver. When the caregiver is the spouse, that person takes on a predominantly caring role in the relationship and receives less comfort and security from their loved one. The caregiving spouse must somehow relinquish their own need for security and focus exclusively on providing care. For many aging couples who enjoy mutually secure relationships, this transition can often be navigated successfully. Those who enjoy secure attachments have a stable sense of being loved by the other. They do not need to have that love

Guilt and Adult Children

demonstrated to them constantly. With a lifetime of happy, loving memories behind them, they are more emotionally equipped to ride out the deterioration in their partner's health. That's not to say they will not feel the compassionate guilt common to many caregivers. But they will be more able to take that guilt in stride and continue to do what is necessary to care for their loved one.

Those who are not so blessed with a secure attachment to their partner may have more trouble. Spouses who lean toward an avoidant attachment style, discouraging closeness, may resent the demands made on them by the growing care needs of their partner. They are more reluctant to embrace the role of caregiver and may become angered by the increased demands on their time and activities. Perhaps not surprisingly, spouses who have an avoidant attachment style are the quickest to move their partner into institutional care.[32]

Spouses who are more anxiously attached appear to be the ones who suffer with guilt the most. These are the relationship partners who repeatedly need signals of love and caring from their partner. While they may be happy to provide care, they cannot relinquish their own need for it. When they don't receive the comfort they need, they may become anxious and angry or resentful. This is the pattern of ambivalence that leads to guilt and, because that guilt cannot easily be resolved, can descend into depression.

Similar patterns can play out when the caregiver is an adult child. Here, there is more of an attachment role reversal whereby the adult child no longer gains comfort and security from their parent and instead must become the provider of care for the parent. How well the adult child and their parent manage this role reversal depends a lot on the history of their adult relationship. As in any relationship, both child and parent have played a role in that history.

The relationship pattern between parents and their adult children that is established in the children's early adulthood can reemerge in the later stages of the parent–adult child relationship when the parents need more care. Parents and adult children who have developed a mutually rewarding relationship can manage the changing needs of the parent better. The children are more open to their changing role in the relationship and are happy to spend more time and effort looking after their parent's care needs. As a result, the parents have less reason to push their children to help. Inevitably, the adult children, like Shannon, will experience pangs of guilt, but this guilt is relatively superficial and does not impact their mental health.

In contrast, parents and adult children who have a more uncomfortable history may have difficulty navigating the changing care needs of the parent. The adult children may resist getting involved in their parent's lives. Some parents, particularly those who are generally anxious in their relationships, may use guilt induction to try to impose filial obligations on their adult children as a tactic to gain their attention and support.[33] This tactic arouses the old frustrations that children had when their parents tried to exert control over them as teenagers and young adults. They remain trapped in an ambivalent dynamic. While they still love their parent, they may feel resentment at having to respond to the parents' demands. Then, when it comes time for the adult child to step up and assume the role of primary carer for their parent, this role may be undertaken with greater reluctance. The adult child ends up in a place where their parent needs regular care and attention, but their gut reaction from the history of the relationship is to resist and resent the control their parent is having over their lives.

This relationship dynamic is the origin of the ambivalence that results in the kind of caregiver guilt that can become overwhelming. The carer feels guilty for feeling resentful and for not being a dutiful child to their parents in their time of need. This is not the momentary pang of guilt that comes from a particular minor event, like Shannon worrying that she didn't take her mother out for ice cream. It is guilt from a persistent, lifelong pattern that colors the whole relationship between the parent and child. With the weight of this lifetime pattern of relating behind it and the pressure of the constant need to provide care, it is not surprising that the adult child's guilt can sometimes lead to severe mental health consequences.[34]

What, if anything, can be done for those caregivers who are at risk of descending into depression from their caregiving responsibilities? The first important step is to recognize that it is the ambivalence in the relationship and the resultant guilt that generate much of the caregiver's negativity. Once this recognition has occurred, the guilt can be targeted by counseling intervention. In a recent clinical trial, a team led by Andrés Losada in Madrid, Spain, found that helping caregivers to recognize their resentment and guilt toward their aging loved one and then reframing that guilt as a natural product of the demands of caregiving helped to reduce their depressive symptoms.[35] An important part of this reframing is to see the current state of the relationship on its own terms and not as a continuation of a lifelong pattern of control. The senior needs care, and the best person to provide it, at least before intensive institutional care is required, is the family member. The senior's need for care is not a continuation of the old dynamic in which the parent was trying to control the child. That phase of the relationship needs to be left in the past.

A second part of the reframing is to recognize that it is perfectly understandable to experience anger toward the parent, especially if they push certain buttons when they show their need. Feeling angry is not a reaction to feel guilty about. Caring for a senior is stressful work, and it will certainly interfere with other goals and interests. So, accept that anger is a reasonable reaction to a tough situation. This therapeutic approach might be seen as employing forgiveness to overcome the guilt. Maybe you could even call it a double dose of forgiveness—forgiveness of the parent for their frustrating tendency to be controlling and forgiveness of oneself for feeling angry about that control.[36]

As we know by now, guilt arises when there is perceived damage to a relationship. As children grow into adolescence and early adulthood, few child-parent relationships are free of conflict. Conflict almost inevitably emerges as children seek to establish their own identities distinct from their family of origin. And so, guilt is commonplace in the experience of both parents and their maturing children. This guilt is heightened when parents attempt to impose their own vision of how their children should make important life choices. It can be particularly exacerbated when parents employ guilt induction as a strategy to control their children's life choices.

As adults age into frailty, their care falls predominantly to their closest family—spouses, if they are available, and more often their adult children. Guilt in caregivers, whether they are spouses or adult children, reflects the love and empathy that caregivers feel as their loved ones' quality of life deteriorates. It may also grow out of resentment when caregiving demands impact other aspects of everyday life. For some adult children who are called upon to be caregivers for their aging parents, guilt may arise with renewed intensity. In some cases, severe guilt can flow from relationship ambivalence, which may have its roots in the tensions established earlier in the child-parent relationship. These cases demonstrate that mental health can be severely impacted by guilt brought on by the stress of changing and challenging life events. When I was reviewing the research discussed in this chapter, I reflected on my own relationships with my parents and wondered how I might have responded to the challenges of caring for them as they aged. That eventuality never transpired—both my parents died of cancer before they experienced difficulties in caring for themselves. Nevertheless, I think there is a good chance that if I had been called on to provide care for my parents suffering with dementia, I might well have experienced the kind of guilt reviewed in this chapter. As we will see next, my mental health was impacted by severe guilt brought on by the stresses of significant changes in relationships. So, let's turn now to review in more detail how and why guilt may go awry to affect mental health in various ways.

Chapter Eight

Guilt Gone Awry

"Tell me what you are feeling right now as you sit in this room with me," Dr. F said, after we had settled into our chairs. His office was a windowless interior room at his hospital practice, dimly lit, and messy with papers, academic journals, and books. Facing me, on a tripod, a small camcorder recorded our therapy session. Dr. F would review the tape afterward for consistency and perhaps share it with colleagues for advice on his clinical interpretation. Being a believer in the value of evidence, I had agreed, despite my reservations about exposing myself in this way, to this collective exploration of my psychic pain.

Dr. F had a kindly and intelligent face, bearded like Sigmund Freud, although I'm sure that was not his intention. He never wore a tie or jacket in my experience, and I appreciated this lack of formality—to me, it was a sign of authenticity and commitment to what matters in the therapeutic relationship. His opening question was the same one he had asked every session since I began a relatively unusual program of therapy called Intensive Short-Term Dynamic Psychotherapy (ISTDP) with him.[1] I had been referred to Dr. F for depressive symptoms—an inability to motivate myself and find joy in my personal life at a time when my mother was dying of cancer and my wife was pregnant with our daughter.

When he had first asked me this question—a pretty simple one—I had groped around for the right words. "I...um...I suppose I'm feeling a bit nervous and unsure; wondering what I am doing here."

"Ok, but you came here for a reason, so if you set aside this uncertainty, tell me what you are feeling."

"Well, I need to know what you are trying to get at; what exactly are you asking me to describe?"

I'm an academic psychologist, trained to analyze and dissect the intentions behind words and actions. My default mode is to try to understand, not to feel. Dr. F was not really concerned with this reaction to his request, but he recognized the need to indulge me so as to build our relationship—the so-called therapeutic alliance.[2] He followed my tangent for a short while before abruptly bringing me back to his project.

"So, what is the feeling in your body as you sit here with me?"

"I don't really know. I guess I feel numb."

We didn't get too far in that first session using ISTDP, but the pattern was established. Every time we met, Dr. F would direct me to focus on my feelings; I would deflect as best I could.

After a few months of regular sessions, we had made some progress, and I learned to go directly to feelings when he asked his opening question.

"I'm feeling a bit tense today; I can feel some nausea in my stomach."

"Concentrate on these feelings. Tell me what they feel like."

I gripped the arms of the chair tightly. Although I knew that we needed to focus on feelings, I still found it difficult to open up unreservedly, and I resented Dr. F for pushing me.

"There's tension in my arms and in my chest."

"What happens if you let that feeling grow? Don't resist it."

I closed my eyes and tried to focus on the tension. I could feel it growing, getting tighter. There was an anger brewing. "I'm starting to feel angry," I said.

"What does that anger want to do? If you stop resisting it, what will it do?"

I resisted—I couldn't help it. "It feels too rigid; it's binding me tightly."

"But if you don't let it bind you, if you let it loose, what will it do?"

Finally, I was able to cough up the answer: "It wants to lash out."

"How does it want to lash out? What does it want to do?"

I couldn't respond.

Dr. F. persisted. "If you let that anger have its way, what will it do?"

I squeezed out the answer: "It makes me want to hit you, to beat on you with my fists."

Dr. F. was unperturbed, and his voice remained calm. "So, you beat on me with your fists, and then what does the anger want to do?"

Dr. F's mild reaction encouraged me. "It keeps going. I keep beating on you."

"Where on my body are you beating me?"

"On your stomach, your sides, your shoulders."

"Tell me where you are as you beat me."

Somehow, I had been transported to the front garden of my childhood home in my imagination, and I was startled to see that I had picked up a large stick and was using it to hit Dr. F. I told him this.

"So, you hit me with the stick. And then what happens?"

What happened was that I was no longer in control. My imagination had taken over, and I was a passive observer of what was now a violent movie, with me as the lead character. My voice was starting to break as I said, "I beat you repeatedly and knock you to the ground unconscious."

"So, you have knocked me to the ground. I want you to look at the face of the person on the ground. Look into the eyes. Tell me whose eyes they are."

I looked with my mind's eye at the body and the face and eyes. Suddenly, it was not Dr. F at all; it was my mother. I had violently beaten my mother. As I looked into her brown eyes, I saw that they were not really looking back at me. I became again the little boy that so desperately craved her love and attention. I was shocked and I collapsed into uncontrollable sobbing. The tension completely left my body. I cried and cried—it took some minutes to gradually subside.

As my crying came to an end, it was time for the postmortem. Dr. F explored with me my feelings toward my mother and asked me about any memories that came to mind. I told him about the incident at the bus stop on my first day of school and what my mother said to me as she dragged me home.

This experience—what would be called a "breakthrough"—happened several times during my therapy with Dr. F.* After these

---

* I should perhaps emphasize that I am not by nature a violent person. These episodes of violent fantasy released during ISTDP are more akin to dreams. Through the therapy, previously unconscious anger is brought to the surface of consciousness and seeks expression in imagination. Part of that expression is what the anger might do. Once the fantasy has occurred, it can be analyzed and understood through the therapeutic process.

episodes, I was able to recall different events from my very early childhood, times when I needed maternal comfort and my mother was unwilling or unable to deliver it. Like all young children, I loved my mother intensely, but I came to realize that her tendency to demand maturity and independence from me even when I was very young, frustrated me and made me angry at her. I could not express that anger for fear of losing her love, so instead, I adopted *her* anger, turned it inwards, and blamed myself for having those feelings toward her. This guilty emotional dynamic was established very early in my life, before I was able to reflect on it rationally, and it became an unconscious and automatic response whenever I felt frustration or anger toward loved ones. In this way, a pattern of relating to others, particularly those whom I am close to, was set in motion for the rest of my life. Whenever I was angry at a loved one, I would inhibit that anger and turn it against myself, which led to the depressive symptoms. It reached a climax during that period in my life because my mother was dying ("abandoning" me for the final time) and because my wife's pregnancy and the impending birth of our daughter required me to set aside my personal passions—in particular, a singular focus on my academic work—to devote my attention to them.

My experience in therapy revealed to me how insidious unconscious guilt can be and convinced me that the kinds of claims made over the last hundred years by psychodynamically oriented psychotherapists about the importance of unconscious guilt in mental health had a solid basis in truth. In my case, the experience of ISTDP was truly profound. ISTDP is an offshoot of psychoanalysis developed and refined by Habib Davanloo, an Iranian-born psychiatrist based at the Montreal General Hospital and McGill University. Like traditional Freudian psychoanalysis, ISTDP assumes that present-day psychological troubles originate in the dynamics of the early childhood relationships between the client and their attachment figures, most often their mother and father. In contrast to traditional psychoanalysis, or "talk therapy," in which the therapist allows the client to explore the thoughts and feelings they have toward loved ones, and then offers interpretations, ISTDP focuses on the emotions that the client experiences. This approach yields substantial benefits for a range of psychological conditions within much shorter time frames than traditional psychoanalysis.[3]

Guilt Gone Awry

The therapist's role in ISTDP is to develop a relationship of trust that opens a channel for the client to reconnect with their ambivalent feelings toward significant people in their life. The catharsis of experiencing these early, unconsciously held emotions is important because it brings them to awareness in a way that may never have happened before. The client sees the emotional dynamics of their significant relationships in a new way and is also able to see how the patterns of relating to others in the present reflect those patterns established early in life.

But catharsis alone is not enough for healing. The therapist also helps the client develop a perspective from which to look back on these early feelings, as well as to recognize them and manage them in the present. We have seen in earlier chapters that guilt is relieved by forgiveness and reconciliation. When I became aware during therapy of my childhood anger at my mother and the guilt I felt for having this anger, I was able to reflect on those feelings in a new way. I saw that my mother's reaction *was* at times overly harsh and that my childish frustration *was* justified. I was a young child whose emotional needs were not met. I loved my mother and at the same time hated her for rebuffing my needs. But these events had occurred forty years in the past, and my mother was now close to death. These were not matters that I needed to rehash with her. Instead, as I reflected on my childhood in this way, I was filled with empathy for the child that I had been. I cried again in sadness for my younger self and forgave myself for those childish feelings.[4]

The emotional release achieved through these breakthroughs in therapy transferred seamlessly into everyday life. My depression was the downstream product of the original unconscious anger and guilt I felt toward my mother, made particularly salient as she was leaving me for the final time. As I became able to bring these feelings to light, and forgive myself for having them, my depression gradually melted away. I became able to recognize the emotional signs of unconscious guilt in my everyday relationships, and while I may not have perfected the art of managing that guilt, I have found that it does not seep perniciously into my emotional life anymore.

My therapy for depression opened my eyes to the way guilt can serve as the engine of mental distress. My guilt in connection with my mother was established long before I developed autobiographical memory—the type of memory that allows us to link up the events of our lives into a personal narrative or story. Because those events, even before the school bus incident, weren't part of my conscious memories, the guilt persisted in a kind of Precambrian stratum in my mind and continued to influence my life. When I felt angry with someone I loved, the unconscious guilt dampened my feelings, and I became depressed. For me, resolving that guilt was profoundly important.

Throughout this book, I have argued that guilt is generally an adaptive emotion—it plays an important and valuable role in managing our social lives—but that it can also, under certain circumstances, lead us astray. Sometimes, this misdirection may be relatively minor and right itself naturally. But, sometimes, guilt leads us so far astray that our psychological health is deeply affected.

When I discussed the nature of guilt in Chapter 1, I suggested some different ways that guilt can go astray, and in the rest of this chapter, I'm going to concentrate on three of them, which can lead to different forms of psychopathology. First, the emotional balance of the "guilt cocktail" of empathy for the other, fear of relationship loss, and self-directed anger can be upset such that one emotional element dominates. Perhaps the worst type of imbalance is an extreme form of remorseful guilt—when self-directed anger or remorse overwhelms the other emotional components. If guilt is felt primarily as anger against the self and it becomes all-consuming, then depression can ensue. This was the engine of my own depression and is common in many forms of depression. Second, we have seen that others can take advantage of a relationship partner's tendency to feel guilt and use it for manipulation. In very close relationships, such as families, this pattern can lead to pathology in some situations. Certain forms of eating disorder, most notably anorexia, may be the result of this kind of guilt induction. Third, when guilt is unresolved because a relationship partner is no longer available for the guilt to be dissipated through forgiveness and reconciliation, then the guilt may persist and can become chronic. Post-traumatic stress disorder often reflects this kind of pathology of guilt.

Guilt Gone Awry

Depression

Since the earliest days of conceptualization of depression as a form of mental disorder, guilt has been implicated.* In the current *Diagnostic and Statistical Manual of Mental Disorders* (DSM-5), used as the primary tool for the diagnosis of mental health conditions, guilt appears as one of the criteria in diagnosing a major depressive disorder.[5] But the role of guilt in depression is complicated. There is now lots of evidence that the simple tendency to feel guilt is not associated with depression.[6] If everyday experiences, such as the guilt we may feel over thoughtless gossiping, brought on depression, life would be unmanageable. Research studies using the TOSCA measure we discussed in Chapter 4 have found that people who are more prone to feeling guilt do not show more depressive symptoms than those who are less prone to guilt. From everything we have seen in this book, this should not be a surprise. Overall, feeling guilt is a healthy response in that it motivates us to try to repair relationships we may have harmed. But there are forms of guilt that are not so healthy. The DSM-5 refers to "feeling worthless or excessive/inappropriate guilt," and it is these forms of guilt that we need to understand better.

As we saw in Chapter 2, feeling worthless is related to feeling shame, which tends to occur when the person concentrates their negative feelings on themselves rather than on their action and its effect on others. The person experiencing shame thinks of themselves as unlikable or unlovable and tends to shy away from relationships and from trying to find solutions to relationship problems. They think that nothing they can do will help. This way of thinking inevitably depresses mood and, over time, may lead to clinical depression. Many research studies have shown that feelings of shame or being prone to shame are more strongly

---

* Although guilt clearly plays an important role in depression, it is important to recognize that "depression" is a term covering quite a broad spectrum of psychological distress. There are those for whom depression is chronic, always in play, even if it waxes and wanes over time. For others suffering from bipolar disorder, depression is one pole of a cycle that transitions back and forth with bouts of mania. There is good reason to believe that bipolar disorder and, in some cases, chronic depression are the result of biological factors and are best treated pharmacologically, although psychotherapy can also be helpful.

connected to depression than being prone to simple guilt. June Tangney and her colleagues used the TOSCA measure to assess degrees or levels of susceptibility to guilt and shame in a large sample of undergraduates.[7] They also measured the level of depressive symptoms in the sample using the most common assessment, the Beck Depression Inventory (BDI). Their results showed that the more participants felt shame, the more likely they reported symptoms of depression.

Whereas the tendency to experience healthy guilt is unrelated to depression, there are other forms of guilt implicated in depression. The DSM-5 refers to "excessive/inappropriate" guilt. This label is a bit vague in that it does not explain exactly what it means for guilt to be "inappropriate" or how much guilt is too much. To bring a bit more clarity to these issues, Carlos Tilghman-Osborne and his colleagues at Vanderbilt University designed a new measure for children and adolescents, called the Inappropriate and Excessive Guilt Scale (IEGS), to test whether respondents tended to feel normal or abnormal levels of guilt, and whether their scores were connected to depression.[8] They included twenty-four hypothetical scenarios for participants to judge. Here is one example:

You overhear your parents arguing but cannot make out any of the words they are saying.

- How much would you think: It's probably my fault they are arguing?

- Would you feel sick to your stomach because it is your fault?

Respondents were to rate each response on a scale of 1 to 3. In this example, the first response assesses inappropriate guilt and the second response assesses excessive guilt. The researchers tested children and adolescents from seven to sixteen years taken from the general population. Interestingly, there did not seem to be any difference in how participants responded to the inappropriate guilt and the excessive guilt options, perhaps because the distinction was too subtle, so I will just refer to this kind of guilt as "inappropriate." When the researchers examined the connection between scores on the IEGS and the scores on a measure of depression, they found that overall, the higher the respondents scored on inappropriate guilt, the more they showed indications of depression. However, this picture was complicated by age differences in the results. When the researchers looked at age differences, they found that inappropriate guilt *declined* with age but that the relation between depression scores and inappropriate guilt *increased* with age. In other words, it seems to be normal for younger children to show more inappropriate guilt than adolescents. However, when adolescents do show inappropriate guilt, they are more likely to experience depression. This finding helps to explain the general finding that depression is relatively rare in younger children, but increases markedly as children transition into adolescence and becomes a serious mental health concern for many adults.

One particularly destructive form of inappropriate guilt is "victim guilt." Those who have been victims of abuse, whether physical, sexual, or emotional, often experience depressive symptoms as a consequence. Such symptoms can range in severity and, in the most extreme circumstances, can result in self-harm and suicide. A study by Marcin Sekowski and his colleagues of adolescents between twelve and seventeen years of age who were inpatients in an American psychiatric facility for suicidal tendencies revealed the links between abuse, guilt, depression, and self-harm.[9] The majority of these adolescents had been admitted to hospital for severe depressive symptoms, and a significant number reported previous suicide attempts. The patients were asked to report on whether they had been physically ("people in my family hit me so hard that it left me with bruises or marks"), emotionally ("people in my family called me things like 'stupid,' 'ugly,' or 'lazy'"), or sexually abused ("someone tried to touch me in a sexual way or to make me touch them"). They were also asked to report on their shame and guilt and to complete the BDI to measure their levels of depression. Finally, they were asked to respond to a questionnaire that assessed the degree to which they experienced "suicidal ideation," or the tendency to have thoughts about committing suicide. The researchers' overall idea was that the shame and guilt associated with the abuse were the emotional pathways that lead to depressive symptoms and, in turn, suicidal thoughts. The results of the study showed clear patterns. Shame and guilt were strongly related to negative mental health status—the more shame and guilt the adolescents reported, the more depressed they were and the more likely they were to report suicidal thoughts.

Abuse was shown to be a clear cause of both shame and guilt. But when it came to analyzing the impact of different forms of abuse, a more nuanced pattern of results was found. From their study, it appears that emotional forms of abuse were more likely to lead to shame rather than guilt, whereas sexual abuse was more likely to lead to guilt rather than shame. This pattern is interesting in that it appears that emotional abuse leads to the victim feeling bad about themselves (shame), whereas sexual abuse leads to the victim feeling bad about what was done to them (guilt).

The idea that we feel guilty about things that are done to us seems counterintuitive. Why should a victim of abuse feel guilty for what someone else did to them? Earlier, I described how, through therapy, I discovered that I felt guilty when I craved my mother's comforting attention and became angry at her when I did not receive it. There are psychological parallels between my early experiences and those of people who have experienced abuse. Although I would not want to classify my experience as genuinely traumatic, because I don't want to devalue the impact of child abuse or sexual violence; nevertheless, like me, many victims of trauma feel guilty in reaction to what was done to them. Again, this guilt seems counterintuitive because of the way guilt is usually framed—in terms of transgressions of moral or legal rules. If someone does something morally wrong—say physically or sexually abusing their child—surely *that* person should feel guilty, not the victim. But this is not how guilt works. As we have seen throughout this book, guilt is stimulated by the recognition that a relationship has been damaged. And most forms of abuse are perpetrated by people with whom the victim has a close relationship. When we reframe guilt as the emotional signal that a relationship has been damaged, then victim guilt makes perfect sense. It is natural for victims, particularly children, to fear that they may in some way be responsible for damaging the relationship and thus also responsible for what was done to them. The problem is that because the victim holds no responsibility for the damaged relationship and thus has nothing to make amends for, their feeling of guilt cannot be put into service to heal the relationship, and so it persists, leading to chronic self-blame and poisoning the mental health of the victim.

If guilt is implicated in depression, then what therapeutic approaches are recommended? Depression is sometimes classified under the more general heading of "internalizing" disorders of mental health. Internalizing disorders are those in which the person's mental torment is turned inwards against the self.* Depression may be thought of as a generalized negativity toward the person's own life and their damaged relationships with loved ones. The key to therapy is to bring the guilt to awareness, and, in particular, the self-directed anger and remorse that are driving the depression, and then find alternative ways to think and feel about relationships. For some clients, it is possible to try to identify and correct negative patterns of thought in everyday life, and cognitive behavioral therapy (CBT) is the gold standard treatment in such cases.[10] For others, like me, it can be better to consider the symptoms as the outcome of relationship damage entrenched early in development, which may be better managed primarily through psychotherapy like ISTDP.

Eating Disorders

Eating disorders constitute a category within the DSM-5 that includes different conditions unified by abnormalities in eating patterns.[11] The category of eating disorders includes conditions in which food intake is restricted in some way—most commonly anorexia nervosa and bulimia nervosa—as well as conditions in which food intake is excessive—such as binge eating and overeating leading to severe obesity—or otherwise odd, such as pica, which is a compulsion to eat nonfood materials like dirt or hair. Although these disorders are grouped together by virtue of them all involving abnormal eating, they have different causes and treatments. Of all the eating disorders, anorexia nervosa is generally the most serious because it is characterized by self-starvation, leading to severe weight loss as well as other health issues, and even death in extreme cases. The DSM-5 criteria for eating disorders make no reference to guilt, but instead focus on the symptoms directly tied to

---

* Internalizing disorders are contrasted with the so-called externalizing disorders, where the symptoms are expressed outwardly, often against others. Externalizing disorders include conditions such as aggression and violence, antisocial behavior, hyperactivity, and destructive behavior such as pyromania.

the abnormal eating behavior. Nevertheless, research on these disorders over the last forty years or more has regularly pointed to a role for guilt.*

Emily Frank of Harvard University appears to have been the first to explicitly study the tendency of women with eating disorders to feel guilt and shame in connection to eating.[12] In a sample of undergraduates, she found that women diagnosed with an eating disorder reported much higher levels of shame and guilt associated with eating than women with depressive symptoms but no eating disorders. Both these groups reported more shame and guilt than women who reported no eating disorder or depression.

Again, as we saw with depression earlier, the picture is complicated with respect to the contributions of guilt and shame. We would not necessarily expect healthy guilt to be associated with an eating disorder, and, indeed, it appears not to be when assessed by measures such as the TOSCA.[13] Some studies have suggested that shame is related to eating disorders, but the clearest finding seems to be that both guilt and shame specifically in connection with eating are the strongest predictors of eating disorder symptoms. The link between guilt and shame and disordered eating applies not only to restricted eating problems like anorexia and bulimia, but also to binge eating.[14] The message from these studies is that for those who have disordered eating, food tends to be associated with guilt and shame.

Where does this connection between food and guilt come from? The roots of the association appear to be in the tendency to link feelings of self-worth with appearance, particularly of the body. Slim is seen as good, overweight as bad. For some women, and a smaller proportion of men, body image contributes to an inordinate degree to self-confidence and self-esteem. The message for women that being slim makes one a worthy and desirable person is pervasive throughout our culture. Failure to attain those perceived body image standards can lead women in particular to feel shame and guilt over their eating habits, whether or not their eating is excessive, restrictive, or even healthy and balanced.

---

* In general, women are about three times more likely than men to be diagnosed with an eating disorder. The reasons for this difference are not completely clear and may include biological causes as well as psychological factors. Because of this gender difference, there are many more studies of eating disorders in women than men.

People who are preoccupied with their body image risk becoming stuck in a vicious cycle of dysfunctional food-related behavior and negative emotion. Failure to attain their body image goals leads to shame over their appearance. This negative feeling of shame can have inconsistent results. On the one hand, it motivates restrictions on food intake through dieting or purging. On the other hand, for those who gain comfort in food, it can lead to binge eating. In turn, binge eating and failure to stick to the restrictions of a diet result in guilt, which further exacerbates the negativity associated with eating and self-image.

Shame associated with body image and guilt associated with bingeing or with lack of control over dieting can often be treated with psychotherapies such as CBT.[15] The therapist explores with the client the feelings associated with their body image and eating. The main goal of the therapy is to interrupt the self-defeating patterns of thought, such as blaming oneself for bingeing or breaking a diet, that maintain the eating disorder. At the same time, shame is targeted by working on the role that body image plays in self-esteem, and refocusing the client's thought toward other areas of positive self-image. CBT is now considered to be the most effective treatment option for bulimia nervosa and binge eating disorder in particular. The contemporary movement to present more realistic body images in popular culture along with a "no body shaming" message is likely also to be a valuable societal corrective in this regard.

The idea that guilt and shame over body image can result in disordered and unhealthy eating habits by perpetuating patterns of dieting, binge eating, and purging seems bad enough, but sometimes restrictive eating can reach a truly pathological and life-threatening extent. Indeed, anorexia nervosa has the highest mortality rate of all psychiatric conditions. The simple idea that a poor body image primes the person to feel guilt about eating seems to lose its authority when the person acquires such a disordered body image that they believe they are too fat even when they are clearly emaciated and have lost all body fat and even most muscle. Here, it seems we may need a different explanation. In such cases, the eating disorder itself is a symptom of a deeper pathology.

In her powerful introduction to anorexia, *The Golden Cage*, Hilde Bruch described with the help of illustrations drawn from many case histories, the classic pattern of an anorexic adolescent or young adult and her family.[16] The typical family of the severely anorexic girl is what is known as "enmeshed." Enmeshed families have strong internal bonds and may appear intimate and trouble-free from the outside. The child, and this is particularly true for girls, feels a strong sense of responsibility toward her parents, most often her mother. At the same time, the parents signal to their child that they are reluctant to allow their child to engage fully with the world outside the family. In the enmeshed family, the child is held hostage emotionally within the confines of the family's needs ("the golden cage" was a term used by one of her patients). The most commanding responsibility is to the family and particularly the mother herself, so much so that the child is often not aware of having her own desires or interests other than those prescribed for her. She may also become fearful of the change in social position as sexual maturity and associated bodily changes beckon. As the girl reaches adolescence, the time when the call of independence from the family typically becomes loudest, she becomes conflicted over the need to continue to care for her parents emotionally, and conform to their interests for her, and the desire and external expectation to explore her own development as a person. Bound by her intense love of her family and afraid to rebel, her need for independence and autonomy comes out as the rejection of that element that her family has provided since birth: nourishment. In describing what she terms the "anorexic stance," Bruch concludes, "These stories of tragic long-term invalidism suffered by these women illustrate that anorexia nervosa is…much more than dieting gone wild. Its true beginning is in the child's passive participation in life.…The relationship to parents appears superficially to be congenial; actually it is too close, without necessary separation, individuation, and differentiation."[17]

Bruch describes the family context for anorexia to arise, but building on her work, Michael Friedman showed how unconscious guilt operates within the context of the enmeshed family to become the engine of the eating disorder.[18] Friedman argues that the anorexic holds unconscious guilt, which may have been established very early in life, for wanting to pursue their own goals, rather than the ones established for them by the family. This guilt comes, of course, from the love the child has for the parents and the deep-rooted concern that by not conforming to their parents' wishes, they will harm their relationship with their parents. And unfortunately, as Friedman says, "these beliefs are encouraged by parents who convey to their children an inaccurate sense of their ability to affect the quality of their parents' lives." In this family system, the parents play a key role in inducing the guilt that their child feels. In illustration, Friedman presents a letter from a mother to her daughter, who had left their town to attend college on the East Coast of the US. After receiving the letter, the daughter returned home and became anorexic shortly after.

> *It's hard to believe that just 19 years ago you were in my tummy next to my heart. Although you are no longer in my tummy you will always remain next to my heart.... Your father misses you very much, too, and wonders about your unconcern for him. He works so hard to provide the material comforts we all enjoy and which, I might add, have enabled you to have this extended vacation in B. He too would love to take a vacation. I wish he had—then there would not have been the money to support your extensive absence and I would not have to write this painful letter.... Let us know what your plans are and when we can expect you home.*
>
> *Hugs and hugs, Mommy*[19]

This family systems analysis of the origins of anorexia points to three important elements of a therapeutic approach. First, and most critically, the sufferer's weight must be established in a range that is not actively life-threatening. Then, ideally, the family as a whole needs to be engaged to explore and hopefully resolve the relationship dynamic by which the parents enable the guilt in their child. Importantly, the tendency to induce guilt in the sufferer needs to be addressed and curtailed. Finally, the sufferer needs to undergo personal psychotherapy to bring to the surface the emotions, such as anger and guilt, that have been turned inwards onto the self. If all three components can be carried out, then the anorexic sufferer may recover a healthy lifestyle.[20]

Post-Traumatic Stress Disorder

Post-traumatic stress disorder (PTSD) is a condition of severe emotional distress following exposure to intense traumatic events, in particular those involving "death, threatened death, actual or threatened serious injury, or actual or threatened sexual violence."[21] PTSD can occur after the sufferer is the victim of trauma, causes trauma themselves, or witnesses trauma in some way. The critical aspect of PTSD is that, because of the exposure, the sufferer experiences repeated uncontrollable, intrusive reminders of the traumatic event in nightmares or waking flashbacks. This continual reexposure is accompanied by a range of distressing emotions, including fear, horror, anger, guilt, and shame. Given the unpredictability of the intrusions, the sufferer may remain in an almost constant state of arousal, try to avoid any situations that might trigger a flashback, and have trouble concentrating and sleeping, leading to serious negative impacts on their everyday life. Not surprisingly, PTSD can become intolerable and is often associated with other mental health problems, including depression, anxiety, substance abuse, and risk of suicide, which can all be seen as downstream effects of the emotional impact of trauma.

The clinical concept of PTSD was first formalized in 1980 in the third edition of the DSM through the advocacy of psychiatrists and support groups working with veterans, holocaust survivors, and survivors of sexual violence. All these groups represented patients who had been exposed to traumatic conditions outside the range of normal experience—war, concentration camps, rape—and were showing the symptoms described earlier. Similar symptoms may also sometimes appear in survivors of natural (earthquakes, hurricanes, etc.) and manmade (major traffic accidents, airplane crashes, etc.) disasters in which shock, severe injury and death have occurred. Because of exposure to such events, first responders, such as police officers, firefighters, and emergency medical personnel, experience PTSD at a higher rate than the general population. Even those who are largely witnesses to such harms, such as journalists covering war or catastrophes, are more likely to suffer from PTSD than the average person.

An important issue in understanding the nature of PTSD is to recognize that while it is essential that some trauma has occurred for a patient to receive a PTSD diagnosis, not all those who are exposed to the trauma develop PTSD. This fact points to the need to identify psychological factors that contribute to the onset of PTSD. What characterizes those individuals who develop PTSD after experiencing trauma? One key psychological factor that has been implicated is guilt.

Let's look at some of the different ways in which sufferers respond to trauma with guilt.

The first form of guilt to be identified in PTSD was survivor guilt. Survivor guilt occurs when a PTSD sufferer has survived a traumatic event that took the life of, or severely injured, another person to whom the survivor was close. Survivor guilt was first articulated clearly by William Niederland in the 1960s in the context of the clinical symptoms of concentration camp survivors and other victims of Nazi persecution.[22] Niederland describes how one particular concentration camp practice—the selections—primed survivor guilt. The selections involved choosing prisoners for execution, often to meet quotas of extermination provided by the SS. Those to be executed were usually the weakest or otherwise of least value to the camp leaders, and prisoners, therefore, tried to find ways to signal their health or value. As Niederland recounts,

> One patient survived because at the first selection when everyone had to indicate his occupation, he promptly said he was a carpenter. His brother-in-law, standing next to him, could not bring himself to lie, and was incinerated. A woman patient I examined attributed her survival to the fact that she stuck rags into her mouth each time the selections took place, giving her face a round and healthy appearance, while in reality she was hollow-cheeked and at the end of her strength.[23]

Years later, those patients were almost paralyzed by the repercussions of their trauma and racked by guilt for how they had found a way to survive the concentration camps when so many of their friends and loved ones had been murdered.

Survivor guilt can cover a range from purely existential guilt to what we might call "rationalized" guilt. In the case of existential guilt, the sufferer is simply reacting to the fact that their relationship has been broken—they survived while a loved one perished. But more often, perhaps, the guilt that accompanies the simple fact of survival provokes the survivor to start to look for reasons why they survived and others did not. Did they do all that they could to protect the other? Did the one prisoner condemn his brother-in-law to die by lying about his occupation to evade selection? Such thought patterns are irrational, but they become ruminative and serve to perpetuate the guilt that the survivor feels without ever leading to a resolution—there is no path to restitution and forgiveness.

Not long after Niederland was showing how important guilt was to the experience of PTSD in holocaust survivors, US Army veterans began returning home from the Vietnam War. Many returning veterans had enormous trouble adapting back to civilian life because of the traumas they had experienced, and it quickly became clear that many were suffering intensely from severe PTSD. PTSD-like symptoms had been recognized in war veterans for at least a hundred years, but the experience of Vietnam vets brought renewed focus to this condition. War inevitably exposes those in military service to extreme violence, including death and severe injury, under the most highly stressful conditions. Those on the front line are responsible for causing death and injury to the enemy and sometimes to innocent civilians. They are witness to the injury and death of people close to them, even as they carry some mutual responsibility for protecting their comrades from harm. War is most often experienced in social groups within which there are strong relationships—comrades in arms who are trained to support each other with their lives. These comrades share a particular set of experiences that create unique bonds among them, bonds that are not easily shared with those who have not been through the same training and experiences, such as family members back home. It is easy to see how these conditions create a hotbed for guilt feelings.

In all wars, veterans witness their comrades falling when it could just as easily have been themselves. As a result, like holocaust survivors, they are highly prone to survivor guilt. Veterans commonly report guilt over surviving their comrades and will blame themselves for not being able to save them. However, for these Vietnam veterans, the very real survivor guilt was supplemented by the guilt they often felt about their own acts of violence.[24] Even if by its nature, war entails the killing of enemy military personnel, too often innocent civilians also fall victim. In the guerilla war context of Vietnam, and later in the wars in the Gulf region and Afghanistan, the line between military personnel and civilian was blurred, and US soldiers on the ground often could not know who was which. Too often, soldiers were forced to make split-second decisions about whether someone who looked like an innocent civilian was actually an enemy operative, perhaps a suicide bomber. Mistakes were inevitably made, and these veterans had to live with knowing they had taken the lives of innocent men, women, and children. The double dose of guilt is deeply damaging. In one study of a hundred Vietnam veterans suffering from PTSD,[25] the researchers found that 35 percent of the forty veterans who experienced both survivor guilt and guilt about their own combat actions had made a suicide attempt, whereas of the thirty veterans who did not report either form of guilt, none had made a suicide attempt.

A third form of guilt that we see in PTSD is victim guilt. As we saw in the previous section, this kind of guilt is often associated with depression that can result from physical and sexual violence. These forms of violence, and in particular rape, are also strongly linked to PTSD in that the victim may have highly distressing flashbacks and nightmares about their experience, leading them to avoid situations that remind them of their experience and to become hypervigilant about the possibility of another attack.

Large-scale surveys conducted in the US suggest that at least 75 percent of acts of sexual violence against women are committed by someone who is known to the victim, including current and former husbands and boyfriends, friends, and stepfathers.[26] These are all people with whom the victim has a relationship, sometimes deeply intimate. It is no surprise, then, that even though they are blameless, the victim feels guilt from the obvious damage to their relationship with the perpetrator. This guilt will often lead victims to ruminate on how they might be to blame for their assault. And because PTSD will lead sufferers to avoid reminders of their trauma, sexual violence often negatively impacts women's overall interest in sexual activity. So, even in cases where the perpetrator of the original sexual violence was not their partner, the victim may shy away from sexual activity with their innocent partner, thereby risking relationship difficulties and potentially eliciting even more guilt.

We have seen that many PTSD sufferers feel guilt of various kinds, but does this mean that their guilt is responsible at least in part for PTSD? One can imagine various ways in which guilt and PTSD are linked. Perhaps, feelings of guilt emerge out of the traumatic experience, and then this guilt plays a role in the generation of the symptoms of PTSD—the intense distress, the intrusive thoughts and images, the avoidance of situations that evoke memories of the trauma, the hypervigilance, and so on. Alternatively, perhaps, guilt is a result of these symptoms. Maybe the symptoms lead the sufferer to feel guilty about how they are reacting and the impact of their PTSD on their current relationships. As we saw earlier with women victims of sexual violence, it is likely that the circumstances of PTSD sufferers are complex enough to encompass both these ways in which PTSD and guilt are linked. However, there is good reason to believe that guilt growing out of trauma does play a causal role in generating the symptoms of PTSD. And this has implications for the treatment of PTSD.

An important aspect of PTSD is the way in which traumatic experiences are reexperienced by the sufferer, sometimes in out-of-the-blue flashbacks, in nightmares, or through some kind of cue in the environment. The reliving of the traumatic experience is what maintains the distress, interferes with both waking life and sleep, creates hypervigilance, and causes the sufferer to avoid situations that may provide potential reminders. Reexperiencing the trauma can be caused by environmental circumstances. A rape victim may have a flashback if they visit a bar in which they had a drink with their assaulter, and so they avoid that location. But sometimes, flashbacks and nightmares seem to come out of nowhere, and, in such cases, it is the internal workings of the mind that generate the memory. The sufferer's guilt is an important part of what keeps them dwelling on the traumatic experience. Guilt leads the person to go over in their mind what happened, how they might have contributed to the harm that was caused, what they might have done differently. In this way, the guilt keeps on serving up reminders of the trauma. Without a resolution of the guilt, the impact of the trauma cannot be defused.

Although it was not derived from real PTSD sufferers, there is experimental evidence for this process. Konstantin Bub and Miriam Lommen of the University of Groningen used a guilt-induction procedure to create guilt in a group of student participants.[27] The approach was a bit like the broken toy procedure to induce guilt in young children that we looked at in Chapter 3. The students were brought to the laboratory on two consecutive days by a researcher, ostensibly to participate in a two-part study. One part was an assessment of attitudes toward sustainable behavior. The participants watched a video on sustainable behavior and completed a series of questionnaires. The participants also completed a supposedly independent test of typing skill presented on a computer. During the typing test, the computer crashed, at which point the researcher complained that a lot of valuable data had been lost. For one group of participants, the researcher went on to blame them for how they had responded on the test. A comparison group of students went through the same procedure, but for them, the researcher said the crash happened regularly and it was nothing to do with them. On the second day, the participants returned to the laboratory to complete another set of questionnaires, including a measure of guilt, and were instructed to complete a week-long diary in which they would report on thought intrusions relating to their participation in the study. Finally, after the participants had completed the diary over the subsequent week, they were informed about the real purpose of the study and told that the computer crash was fabricated.

Two important differences were seen between the participants who were blamed for causing the computer crash and those who were not blamed. First, those who were blamed reported higher levels of guilt on the guilt questionnaire than those who were not blamed, so the procedure was successful in creating guilt. Second, according to their diaries, those who had been blamed experienced many more thought intrusions about their experience in the laboratory in the following week than those who had not been blamed. They also reported experiencing much higher levels of distress associated with their memories of their experience. Now, of course, the participants' experience in this experimental guilt induction would not be considered a trauma in any clinical sense, but nevertheless, the experiment shows neatly how guilt can be an engine for subsequent thought intrusions and distress, two of the key elements of PTSD. As we have seen, guilt alerts us to how we have damaged a relationship and motivates us to try to find ways to heal that damage. When healing is not possible, as in real trauma cases and in this experimental case, the guilt just keeps prompting us to no avail and can become chronic.

Understanding guilt as one of the engines of PTSD points to a possible therapeutic path. The National Center for PTSD in the US recommends trauma-focused psychotherapy as the best approach to treating PTSD.[28] Such psychotherapy can include different approaches to turn off the power of guilt to generate PTSD.[29] One is to defuse guilt by correcting faulty ways of thinking about the original trauma. As we have seen, PTSD sufferers often imagine how they might have been at fault for the original tragic events. Those with survivor guilt and victim guilt are especially prone to this kind of faulty "hindsight" thinking. In such cases, the therapist can work on retraining the sufferer's thought patterns so that they understand and accept that feeling guilty does not mean they did something wrong. They are helped to recognize that the guilt they feel comes from the relationship loss or damage, not from their actions.

A second component of therapy aimed at the guilt in PTSD, particularly in those cases where the guilt comes from some harmful act that the sufferer performed, as may be the case with war veterans, is to try to help the sufferer find a way to make amends or restitution and achieve forgiveness. As we have seen, making amends entails a genuine feeling of remorse and a sincere apology. Even if those harmed by the sufferer's action are not in a position to accept an apology and grant forgiveness, offering it can be a critical step toward being able to forgive oneself.

I have made a strong claim in this chapter: that guilt is the engine that generates the psychic pain of a variety of severe internalizing kinds of psychopathology. The three main conditions I have described—depression, eating disorders, PTSD—sit in quite different places in the organization of the DSM-5, but for each, guilt is an important source of negative emotion, thought, and behavior. The forms of guilt, and the way the guilt comes about, vary. But in each case, the role of guilt as an alert that relationships have been harmed is clear. In many cases, guilt has its roots in the dynamics of family relationships. Sometimes, this guilt originated in early childhood and then resides in the unconscious emerging as emotional and behavioral dysfunctions later in life, when echoes of the past are felt in significant relationships in the present. Guilt may also arise because of extreme adverse circumstances in adulthood when significant relationships are potentially or actually damaged. In each case, the guilt persists because there is no easy way for the sufferer to relieve it. Self-blame takes over and the guilt poisons the emotional life of the sufferer. The resulting distress can lead to misery, self-harm, escape into substance abuse, and even death.

The path to healing comes with recognizing how one's relationships are implicated and then finding ways, if possible, to heal those relationships. And it is highly valuable to have an outside perspective in the form of a therapist to complete this work. Where the damaged relationships are still in place and having their effects, relationship-focused therapy, such as family therapy or couples therapy, can be an effective approach to bringing to light and resolving the guilt. But, sometimes, the relationship partner is no longer available. In those cases, such as my own, a therapist can help one to heal one's *attitude* toward the relationship. For me, it was necessary to work through the elements of my guilt in therapy, and that work was lengthy and tough. Relief came when I could empathize with and forgive my mother for not always providing the attention and care that I needed as a child, and when I could empathize with and forgive myself for the anger, of which I was initially completely unaware, that I felt toward her. When I did this, I could relinquish the self-blame that was causing my depression.

I have concentrated on these three severe forms of psychopathology because, in these cases, unconscious guilt can be crippling. But guilt can play a role in many other lesser forms of psychic pain that detract from living a psychologically healthy life. In all cases, understanding the role of guilt is critical for finding the way out of these forms of psychological confinement. Guilt needs to be recognized for what it is: emotional pain from self-blame for damaged relationships. Then it is critical to gain clear sight of the relationships that have been harmed and one's true role, if any, in causing that harm. Inappropriate patterns of thought that sustain self-blame for damaged relationships must be identified and retrained. Finally, it is essential to move beyond the punishment of self-blame by forgiving oneself for whatever one may have thought or done.

Part II Takeaways

In Part I, we gained the tools for how to think about guilt and its role in our lives. Part II has described some of the many ways in which guilt shows up in our social relationships. Both everyday experience and psychological research demonstrate that guilt is felt most often and most urgently in our communal relationships—the relationships that are characterized by affection and caring. These are the relationships that we value most and that we most want to keep healthy. Guilt is much less prevalent in relationships that are characterized by an exchange orientation.

The core of communal relationships is the family. Some communal relationships are given by birth and others, such as romantic partners and friends, are chosen, but even those that are chosen come to resemble the experience of family. Communal relationships between adults are ideally symmetrically and reciprocally balanced. Both partners equally seek affection from the other and both partners equally provide love and caring for the other. Within these relationships, guilt is an important mechanism for sustaining balance. It alerts us to when the relationship may be challenged and motivates us to cultivate the relationship. But when these relationships lack communal balance, as can be the case when one or other partner has an insecure attachment, then guilt is less effective and, as happens when guilt induction is used for relationship management, can even become counterproductive.

Certain communal relationships are by their nature asymmetrical in that one partner provides most of the care for the other. These relationships are particularly prone to eliciting guilt in the carer because of the perceived risk of harm to the other and to the relationship itself. Parents experience guilt around every corner when it comes to child-rearing. Because young children are especially vulnerable and so dependent on the care their parents provide, the concern that parents feel for their children is like no other. Parental guilt keeps parents focused on providing as much high-quality care as possible. This dynamic benefits children but can be very stressful for parents. Mothers are particularly hard hit when it comes to parental guilt. The unique role they play in parenting and the bond they establish with their children from before birth can prime mothers for a lifetime of guilt. But, despite guilt being a common experience for parents, it often is misplaced. For parents, the best solution to the guilt they feel is to consider whether they need to restore the relationship through apology or restitution. In most cases, of course, the answer is probably no.

As children emerge into adulthood, parents and their children often experience strain in their relationship. Maturing children need to develop an identity that is to some extent independent of their family of origin, and parents need to find a way to maintain support yet relinquish control while their offspring explore their independence. Parental guilt induction in this period can be especially poisonous to the quality of the relationship and can lead to resentment and even rupture of the parent-child bond. The damage to the relationship can have long-term negative impacts on the health of the relationship. But when the transition is handled sensitively, it can lead to a lifelong rich relationship for both parents and their adult children.

As adults age into frailty, they become the ones dependent on the care of others. Those others, whether spouses or adult children, are often faced with a situation in which their caring, no matter how solicitous, cannot stem the ravages of time. Under these circumstances, guilt is difficult to resist, but it can also be dissipated by a realistic assessment of the carer's responsibility. For those adult children whose relationships with their parents may have been marked by ambivalence and resentment, guilt over their reaction to their parents' care needs can become debilitating. Here, the normal response of guilt may tip over into an extreme reaction that can compromise mental health and require counseling intervention.

Despite guilt being a normal and healthy emotion in everyday life, unhealthy forms of guilt are not uncommon. Guilt is implicated in a variety of mental health problems, particularly those that fall within the general category of internalizing disorders. In all these cases, the root of the guilt is real or perceived damage to significant relationships. Pathological guilt can come from an imbalance in the emotional makeup of guilt, or because of excessive guilt induction by loved ones, or because there is no simple path to forgiveness. When unresolved, pathological guilt can lead to a variety of self-punishing reactions, including depression, eating disorders, and PTSD. Therapies that bring the guilt to awareness, reframe it as inappropriate, and allow forgiveness to be experienced can be highly effective in helping those suffering from unresolved guilt.

Part III

Guilt in Society

Chapter Nine

Guilt in Religion

The daylight was beginning to lose its summer vibrancy as we approached the outskirts of the ancient French town we were visiting on our summer holiday. My father had been driving most of the day since we had crossed the English Channel by ferry in the morning. After journeying south along poplar-bordered country roads through fields of sunflowers, we had stopped at a campground to set up our tent before heading to the town. My mother sat in the passenger seat attending to the paper map showing the route my father had worked out. I was in the back seat, squeezed in with my brother and sister, tired after a long day of driving. It was Sunday and we were trying to find our way to the center of the town so we could attend Mass at the Catholic church.

I was perhaps nine or ten, and I remember I was going through a stage of intense religious devotion. I was an altar boy at my local church, and I had told my parents earlier in the year that I was going to become a priest. I believed I could talk directly to God and had a vocation for the Church. Growing up Catholic, I was already deeply familiar with religious guilt, and that day, I was about to get a big jolt of it. As Catholics, we were guided by the catechism of the Catholic Church, which, respecting the third of the Ten Commandments, says: "On Sundays and other holy days of obligation, the faithful are bound to participate in the Mass…unless excused for a serious reason (for example, illness)."[1] Through most of the year, this wasn't a problem. Our family attended the parish church for Mass every Sunday and on other religious holidays, and thereby our obligation was fulfilled. Occasionally, I would miss Mass because I was sick, but this was explicitly allowed in the catechism, so I didn't need to worry. But every year in the summer, we would go on holiday for about two weeks, often in

France, and there, we would have to find a church to attend Mass each Sunday we were away.

My parents were Francophiles as well as devout Catholics, and so the opportunity to attend Mass in different churches or cathedrals every summer was a significant joy. They usually would ensure that we timed our travel as well as our Sunday activities to fit with the hours of Mass at the local church wherever we were staying. But this year, the plans were not quite working out. For some reason, we had chosen to travel on a Sunday, and it had taken us a long time to reach our destination. We set about trying to find our way into the center of town, where there would inevitably be a Catholic church. But the narrow cobblestone streets did not seem to match the map, and the one-way system was obviously an innovation. We ended up driving in circles, unable to find our way closer to the center of town. As the time ticked on, my anxiety increased. If we did not find a church soon, we would break the third commandment and be guilty of a grave sin, which, if I died somehow before making it to confession, would mean eternal banishment from God's side. I could tell my father was stressed as he drove; he was getting impatient with my mother beside him in the front seat as she fought with the folds of the map. But I was getting desperate. I pleaded with my parents to find the way, informing them that we had to get to Mass or risk committing a mortal sin. At that moment, I felt the impending guilt as an anxious churning in my stomach and a dread that I might be doomed. My father, to his credit, did not snap at me, but calmly told me that just as it was not a sin to miss Mass when sick, it was not a sin to miss Mass while lost on holiday. I'm not sure if I really believed him, but I did feel somewhat comforted. After all, the fourth of the Ten Commandments required me to honor my father and my mother. We never did get to Mass that day, but I was content on that occasion to let my father's interpretation of the catechism prevail.

The Ten Commandments

1. I am the Lord your God: You shall not have strange Gods before me	Govern the relationship with God

2. You shall not take the name of the Lord your God in vain

3. Remember to keep holy the Lord's Day

4. Honor your father and your mother Govern relationships with other people

5. You shall not kill

6. You shall not commit adultery

7. You shall not steal

8. You shall not bear false witness against your neighbor

9. You shall not covet your neighbor's wife

10. You shall not covet your neighbor's goods

As a child, I always knew when I was guilty of wrongdoing because Catholicism, like most religions, has such clear rules about it. In religion class in school and in our church on Sundays, we learned these rules, starting with the Ten Commandments. The Ten Commandments lay out fundamental rules for how to lead a good life. The first three concern the relationship with God and the last seven concern relationships with other people.* But we learned that to break any of the rules

---

* I am describing the Catholic version of the Ten Commandments here. The Jewish version reserves the first four commandments for honoring the relationship with God (as does the Protestant version).

was to sin, and to sin was to put us at odds with God. We were drilled on the difference between lesser venial sins and cardinal, or mortal, sins.[2] Venial sins did not put one at risk for eternal damnation. So, even though I knew I had done wrong, I didn't *feel* particularly guilty when I told my mother I had brushed my teeth when I had not. I just made a mental note to bring it up when I went for confession, in the knowledge that the slate would be easily wiped clean.

The mortal sins proscribed by the Ten Commandments were another matter entirely. The risk here was significantly greater. If I should die having committed a mortal sin, and without genuine contrition and absolution, I could well be in for eternal damnation. But fiery images of hell were not what concerned me; it was the prospect of permanent separation from God, the loving father figure who kept us safe.

The commandments that caused me the most worry were the first three in the list; those governing my relationship with God. I knew that the others to do with relationships between people were important, but really, they didn't apply that much to me at that point in my life. I worried constantly that my relationship with God, or with his mortal incarnation, Jesus Christ, was at risk. Maintaining that relationship involved not just doing His will, but also praying to Him nightly. Once I was old enough to say my own prayers, I worried that I wasn't doing a good enough job. I'd kneel at my bed in the evening before sleep and recite the standard prayer to honor Him, the Lord's Prayer: "Our father, who art in heaven…" As I said the words, I monitored myself to ensure I was reflecting on each one appropriately and concentrating through the whole prayer. If my attention wandered, perhaps to think about what had happened at school that day, I'd start again. The guilt I felt about letting my mind wander led me to become more and more scrupulous about what counted as saying the prayer properly. For a period, I was saying the Lord's Prayer up to a dozen times before I was satisfied.

The second commandment required us not to take the Lord God's name in vain. This too required some vigilance and was quite regularly a source of guilt. Standard common British English expletives at the time included, "Oh, God," "Jesus Christ," and "Cor blimey" (derived from "God blind me"). My friends would wield these expletives with alacrity, as if daring God to punish them. Of course, I didn't want to be left out, so I would often join in. But afterward, I felt terrible. Taking the Lord's name in vain was typically the first thing on my list when I went to confession.

As I see it now, my concern with the first three commandments was because they all related to ensuring that my relationship with God was healthy. I kept on God's good side by praying to Him, by respecting His name, and by attending Mass. Because my version of Catholicism was framed almost entirely in terms of this relationship, the feeling of guilt played a prominent role in my religious life. When I was young, I certainly knew when I was guilty of committing a sin, because I knew the rules. But knowing my guilt was only a part of it. I also felt guilt viscerally, as a dreadful weight of negativity that focused my attention on how I had let God down. And it was this *feeling* of guilt, not the knowledge of the transgression, that motivated me to try to do better, to try to get closer to God.

So, how do Catholics resolve their guilt? Fortunately, Catholicism provides a convenient and flexible method for resolving both the risk of losing one's place by God's side and the negative feelings of guilt. The key to avoiding eternal damnation is to repent, and for Catholics, the sacrament of confession is the critical ritual. As a child, I quickly learned that confession was, quite literally, a godsend. It was the opportunity to relieve myself of the accumulated guilt from the sins I had committed and to right my relationship with God. Our parents would take us to church on a Saturday, and we would sit in a row in the pews, waiting for our turn in the confessional. The confessional was a three-part carved wooden structure. The priest was hidden in the center division. When it was my turn, I would enter the confessional through the maroon velvet curtain on one side and kneel beside an ornate grate. The priest would be sitting on the other side of the grate with his ear clearly visible, the receptacle into which I could pour my misdeeds. I would recite the required wording: "Bless me, father, for I have sinned. It has been a week since my last confession, and I have committed these sins, for which I am truly sorry." I would then recount the list of my sins that I had prepared. The priest would say some words in Latin, absolving me of my sins, and let me know my penance, perhaps three Hail Marys and two Our Fathers, appropriately varied according to the length and severity of my list of sins. I would then leave the confessional and return to my place in the pew, where I would say my penance. That was it:

a few minutes, some minor embarrassment, and a profound sense of relief.

As I reflect on my early life as a Catholic, I can see that the relationship with God was really the core of our religious culture. The rules for good behavior as outlined in the commandments and the catechism specified the dos and don'ts of behavior, but the justification for following them was primarily for the sake of one's relationship with God. Although it was never put in quite these terms, being good to others was essentially a means to an end: to live in harmony with God. And that is why when a Catholic commits a sin, the resolution of that guilt is through contrition, confession, and penance paid to God.

Remarkably, in all the years I went to confession, I don't remember the priest ever advising me to apologize to the injured party of my wrongdoing or to attempt reparation. And my parents essentially took the same approach. They never required me to apologize to whomever I might have harmed. If I hurt my younger sister during a fight and made her cry, I could confess that sin and repair my relationship with God by saying two Our Fathers. I could always expunge my guilt by praying to God. When I reflect on how my guilt as a child was managed through religion, I am struck by the almost total reliance on seeking God's forgiveness through prayer.

But I should note that my early experience of sole reliance on forgiveness from God is not universal. Bernhard Schlink recounts this childhood story in his book *Guilt about the Past*: "One evening I asked God to forgive me for hurting my brother or one of my sisters. After the prayer my mother wanted to know if I had asked for forgiveness from the brother or sister themselves. No, I had not done that. She replied that then I had no right to ask God for forgiveness and that God does not grant forgiveness as long as we have not sought it from those we have injured."[3] In fact, Catholic teaching does encourage apology; it just didn't seem to be part of *my* early experience with religion.

Given my own intense experience with religious guilt growing up as a Catholic, I have been interested as an adult in how different religions treat wrongdoing and its resolution. Of course, I never did become a priest. I renounced Catholicism in my late teens as I sought to develop my own personal conscience. A significant impetus for this change in belief was my reading as a teenager about the variety of religions across the world and the different ways that they conceptualize how to lead a virtuous life. It became clear to me that at the core of all religions are some very basic principles about how to treat other people, or, as I would frame it now, how to manage one's social relationships—loving and caring for others, in particular one's family, treating others with honesty and fairness, respecting property, and so on. I reached a point where I couldn't accept that the religion that I happened to have been born into could be the only true one, when there are billions of people of other religions taking the same view of their own religion.[4] This insight led me to think about the commonalities and differences among these religions from the point of view of psychology.

This idea of living life in harmony with God is common to the three main monotheistic world religions—Judaism, Christianity, and Islam—sometimes referred to as the Abrahamic religions, in that they all trace their heritage in some form to the origin story of how God revealed himself to, and then tested, the prophet Abraham (or Ibrahim in Islam). In the West, Abraham is seen as the transition point in human history between a polytheistic and pagan worldview and a monotheistic one. It was Abraham who first put his complete faith in one God and developed a genuine relationship with that God. In so doing, he became the patriarch of God's chosen people, the Jews. Judaism was the first monotheistic religion, dating from nearly four thousand years ago. Christianity evolved directly from Judaism with the ministry of Jesus Christ, who was born a Jew, about two thousand years ago. Finally, Islam dates from just over fourteen hundred years ago, when Muhammad brought a new interpretation of the Judeo-Christian religious tradition to the Arabian peninsula and founded Islam.*

There are important differences between the Abrahamic religions, and over time, multiple sects with differing beliefs and guidelines for moral behavior within each of the three main branches of the Abrahamic religions have evolved. These differences have led to significant conflict throughout the last two thousand years, with multiple wars and

---

* I should perhaps note that the Islamic belief is that the religious tradition stemming from Abraham/Ibrahim was always Islam. Muhammad's contribution was to correct misunderstandings that had been introduced by followers of prior prophets and messengers. So, in the Muslim worldview, both Abraham and Jesus were "Muslims" in that they submitted to God and encouraged their followers to do so as well.

persecutions occurring between believers on different sides. However, as moral systems, all three religions have much in common. All three articulate a code of behavior with a set of rules, which the faithful must observe to live a moral life. These rules have their origins in the Bible and the Ten Commandments. Failing to adhere to the rules means one is guilty of sin, and this guilt needs to be reconciled through contrition and forgiveness. In addition to respecting human relationships, all three religions stress the fundamental importance of securing a strong relationship with God. So, whether one is Muslim, Jewish, or Christian, one's relationship with the one true God is the touchpoint for a moral life.

The importance of the relationship with God in the genesis of religious guilt can be seen by contrasting the Abrahamic religions with the other main group of world religions that developed in Asia, sometimes called the Dharmic religions, including the various denominations of Hinduism and Buddhism. In Dharmic religions, there is no single all-powerful God, who designed the universe to be a certain way and put in place rules for action. Dharmic religions are more naturalistic, in the sense that the universe is believed to have a particular structure within which people can choose a more enlightened path. Choosing a good life is not motivated by the need to keep one's relationship with God healthy, rather it is to ascend to a higher station in life. The role of spiritual leaders is to provide guidance on how to choose the more enlightened path, not to convey the will of God. The concepts of sin and guilt play essentially no role in this religious structure.[5]

Guilt in Judaism

Judaism was the first monotheistic religion in which God is kind and just and urges believers to follow his example,[6] and so marks perhaps *the* critical innovation in the history of the spiritual lives of ancient humans in what we now call the West. In some ways more a culture than a religion, Judaism involves the fundamental overarching theme of escape from oppression by entering a covenant with God, thereby ensuring delivery to a promised land as God's chosen people. This theme was first enacted when Moses led the escape from slavery in Egypt, as described in the book of Exodus in the Old Testament. It played out several times over history, but of course had its loudest echo in the twentieth-century experience of Jews in Nazi Germany, the Holocaust, and the establishment of the modern state of Israel. The cultural narrative of escape from oppression and the idea of a people chosen by God gives Judaism a more communal orientation. Jews see themselves as a collective—a group with a shared history and culture that distinguish them from other peoples. Jews who do not practice Judaism as a religion still often identify culturally as Jews based on this shared heritage.[7] A colleague of mine shared with me that even though he renounced the religious practice of Judaism in his late teens, he still identifies as a Jew some sixty years later. In contrast, I rejected Catholicism at about the same age and have not identified as a Catholic since! Without the shared history and sense of community, it is less common to be converted to Judaism. And so, despite being the original monotheistic religion, Judaism remains relatively small in terms of number of followers, with approximately 15 million adherents worldwide, certainly compared to Christianity and Islam, which share approximately 4 billion members between them.[8]

In Judaism, God is conceived of as a supernatural presence, active in the material world but also transcending it. God is understood to be omniscient, omnipotent, and omnipresent, and this conception of the power of God has carried through into Christianity and Islam. Given God's transcendent nature, Judaism prohibits representations of God. God is not of the material world and so cannot be represented in iconography that reflects that world. Nevertheless, in the Jewish tradition, it is possible to have a relationship with God. Indeed, Abraham's biblical story is in large part about his relationship with God. God spoke to Abraham and tested his faith by seeing whether he would be willing to sacrifice his son, Isaac.[9] In his turn, Abraham questioned God's decision to destroy the city of Sodom for having turned to evil by reasoning that it would be unfair to destroy a whole city if it contained even a small number of righteous people.

In Judaism, the rules of behavior are articulated in the Torah, primarily derived from the first five books of the Biblical Old Testament: Genesis, Exodus, Leviticus, Numbers, and Deuteronomy. The Torah articulates 613 commandments, some of which are requirements to perform an act and others are requirements to abstain from an act. This may seem like a lot to keep track of. However, many of them do not apply to present-day Jews; they have historical religious significance but cannot be followed. Others are legal directives, such as "The court must judge the damages incurred by a goring ox" and "A judge must not pity the murderer or assaulter at the trial." A variety of other commandments cover areas like how to worship and pray to God ("To bless the almighty after eating"), what to eat and what not to eat and how to prepare food ("Not to cook meat and milk together"), and appearance ("Men must not shave the hair off the sides of their head"). Many of the other commandments that do have direct relevance to contemporary life elaborate on the strictures of the Ten Commandments (for example, "Not to curse your father and mother"). There are two broad types of sin that remain relevant to today's Jews: those that affect the relationship with God and those that affect relationships with other people, the latter generally deemed the worse of the two. Three sins are considered more immoral than any others: idolatry, which compromises one's relationship with God, murder, and prohibited sexual relations. It is better to die than to commit these sins.

When a Jew has committed a sin against another person, their guilt can only be resolved by contrition and forgiveness. Contrition involves performing *teshuvah*, which involves a sincere and rigorous self-examination of their responsibility as well as an apology to the victim and an offer of restitution to right any wrong. With an honest *teshuvah*, responsibility for healing the relationship passes from the perpetrator to the victim, who should grant forgiveness. In this way, therefore, the victim takes the final step to heal the relationship with the perpetrator. Sins committed against God, such as eating prohibited food or committing other prohibited acts, must be similarly resolved by performing a *teshuvah*. In this case, the process is more ritualistic and involves recitation of prayers of confession. While this can happen at any time, once a year on Yom Kippur, the Day of Atonement, the community more generally comes together to perform the *teshuvah* and receive forgiveness from God.

That guilt is pervasive in Jewish experience has become something of a stereotype; think of many Woody Allen characters or Howard Wolowitz on *The Big Bang Theory*. Guilt may appear omnipresent in Jewish experience, but it seems to be manifested particularly at two levels of relationships: community and family. There is a strong communal side to Jewish guilt, reflecting the original covenant between

God and the Jews as the chosen people. For example, even if they do not practice their religion, Jews may abide by certain rules of the Torah, such as not eating pork, when in public, even if not in private, to show their respect for their community. It is possible that in the modern day, this sense of communal guilt is also complicated by a form of survivor guilt in association with the Holocaust. Many modern-day Jews in North America can trace a connection to family members who perished in the Nazi concentration camps simply for being Jewish, and as we saw in Chapter 8, personal survival while others died was fertile ground for the growth of guilt.[10]

Guilt within the family is more about person-to-person relationships and particularly parent to child. The stereotypical image of the Jewish mother who constantly makes her children feel guilty if they fail to meet her expectations or filial obligations appears to have its origins in a postwar ethnographic study by anthropology researchers working with Margaret Mead and Ruth Benedict.[11] They interviewed many European-born Jews who migrated to the US. These Jews had experienced deprivation and persecution in Europe and had come to the new world in search of a better life—in particular for their children. The parenting strategy was to convey the message that they had suffered so that their children could be successful, so they had better be! Whether such guilt induction is genuinely more common in Jewish immigrant families compared to other immigrant families is unclear.[12]

Guilt in Christianity

Christianity arose following the ministry of Jesus Christ in about 30 CE. Christ was born a Jew in what is now Israel and so was already a believer in the one true God. His message of love and forgiveness was powerful enough to recruit a significant following but also brought him into conflict with the Jewish elders of the time, who schemed to have him put to death by crucifixion. After his death, his followers spread his teachings throughout the eastern Mediterranean and finally gained traction as the religion of the Roman Empire with the conversion of Emperor Constantine in the fourth century CE. This allowed Christianity to spread widely throughout the Roman Empire, which at the time encompassed the Mediterranean region, Europe, and North

Africa, and then, beginning in the Renaissance, to Asia, Africa, and the newly discovered North and South Americas through colonization and missionary work by European powers. Christianity has fractured into multiple strands over the last two thousand years, and it is not possible to do justice to the many variations that exist. I will focus on the core themes of Christianity with special reference to Catholicism, because that is what I know personally, but also because the little direct evidence we have suggests that Catholics report stronger guilt feelings than other Christian denominations.[13]

For our purposes, there are two important adaptations that the Christian tradition made to Judaism. The first concerns the nature of sin. Guilt is associated with sin in Christianity as it is in Judaism. If one commits a sin, then one is guilty. As we have seen, the catechism of the Catholic Church lays out the rules that determine whether one has sinned in action. This, then, is also an objective approach to guilt. But in Catholicism, this objective guilt is pervasive and inherited. From the time of the apostle Paul (first century CE),[14] Catholicism locates the inclination to sin in the fall from grace, whereby the first humans, Adam and Eve, disobeyed God's command and were banished from the Garden of Eden. Augustine (354 to 430 CE) developed the idea of a natural human inclination to sin into the doctrine of original sin.[15] According to Augustine, all humans carry the guilt of this original sin at birth and need to be cleansed of it through baptism to be able to live in union with God. But they also retain the tendency to be tempted into sin. An important element of this narrative is the idea that Jesus Christ was put on this earth by God to save humans from sin. Christ made the ultimate sacrifice through his crucifixion to atone for the sins of humans and save them from eternal damnation. So, humans need to believe in Christ the savior to be able to resist the temptation of sin.

The other critical difference that really sets Christianity apart from Judaism (and Islam) is the belief that Jesus Christ is God incarnate.[16] During his ministry, Christ did not explicitly refer to himself as God's son on earth.[17] However, this idea became a cornerstone of Christian doctrine during the following two centuries. It is the transformation of Christ from a spiritual, yet still merely human, leader to the incarnation of God that really marks the schism of Christianity from Judaism. Now, God had taken on human form and a face, allowing a different form of worship. Iconography depicting Jesus began to appear even as

Christianity took root in the eastern Mediterranean. Unlike synagogues (and mosques), Christian places of worship became filled with statues and paintings representing Jesus Christ as well as other religious figures. Perhaps most powerful was the symbol of Christ on the cross—God making the ultimate sacrifice so that the guilt of humans could be absolved. From that point on, the believer could imagine a much more personal relationship with God mediated through the image of Jesus Christ.*

An important component of Christianity is that sin is not limited to action; it also reaches into thought. So, I was guilty of a sin when I took the Lord's name in vain, but I was equally guilty if I only thought about doing so. Because God knows one's thoughts, there is no escaping taking responsibility for one's sins if one wants to maintain a strong relationship with God. The combination of human form and godly omniscience creates a powerful mixture. Because sin can happen in thought as well as deed, for the Christian, taking responsibility for one's sin is necessarily a personal project. No one else may know of your sin if it is just a thought. So, you must be willing to take personal responsibility for your sins and seek reconciliation with God through confession.

The resolution of guilt in Christianity involves two main components. The first, as we have seen, is in accepting that Jesus Christ is the savior, who died for the sins of humans. This resolves the original sin that would otherwise prevent a person from entering heaven. The second, as I described earlier, is to participate in the sacrament of confession. Confession requires three acts of the confessor and occurs in the presence of a priest. First, the confessor must express genuine contrition or sorrow for the sins committed. Second, the sins are disclosed. Finally, the confessor is absolved of the sins contingent on completing some penance recommended by the priest. In the Catholic tradition, confession is a personal ritual between the penitent and the priest, but in some Christian faiths, including the Anglican tradition, confession can occur as part of group worship during Mass.

---

* These two differences between Judaism and Christianity underlie the unattributed zinger: "Jews invented guilt; Catholics perfected it."

Forgiveness is a core theme in Christianity. Just as God forgave humanity through the sacrifice of Jesus, so humans must forgive those who have harmed them. The Lord's Prayer, perhaps the most important and often recited prayer in Christianity includes the line: "And forgive us our trespasses, as we forgive those who trespass against us."

Subjective guilt in Christianity appears to be associated less with failing to meet familial or community standards, and more with failing to meet God's standards and thereby compromising that relationship. I think there is good reason to believe that the fundamentally more personal relationship that Christians have with God in the form of Jesus Christ contributes significantly to this difference. As a real human being who is at the same time one with God, Christ provides the potential for magnification of a meaningful person-to-person relationship. Christ acts as an important mediator of the believer's relationship with God. Just as we feel subjective guilt in our relationships with important people in our lives when we harm them, the faithful feel it in connection to their relationship with Jesus Christ. Living with sin means a damaged relationship with Jesus Christ and the risk of a permanent loss of the relationship with God. It is this subjective guilt that provides the motivation to try to avoid sin as well as to seek redemption.

Guilt in Islam

According to the Islamic biographical writings of the Sīrah, Islam has its origins in the revelations of God's will made to Muhammad by the angel Jibreel (known as Gabriel in the Christian tradition). The revelations proclaimed the existence of the one true God in contrast to the polytheistic beliefs of the Arab tribes of the region in what is now Saudi Arabia. Through a combination of military strength and political influence, Muhammad was able to establish and grow a community throughout Arabia that recognized him as the messenger of God. In 630, he made a triumphant entry into the city of Mecca and fulfilled his mission to destroy the pagan idols of the Kaaba and rededicate the site to the one true God. His reformation of the Mecca pilgrimage is still practiced today in the Hajj that all Muslims are obligated to make at least once in their lifetimes.

From this beginning, Islam spread quickly through the Middle East, Asia, North Africa, and into Europe. In the period prior to European colonialism, Islam was the most widespread religion geographically, and today remains the world's second most populous religion after Christianity. Furthermore, more than any other religion in the modern world, it maintains a strong influence on the political and legal organization of many contemporary nations.

In the teachings of Islam, there is only a unitary God—Allah ("the God"). Humans were created to serve God and to submit to God (*Muslim* means "one who submits"). Islam takes the prohibition of idolatry to a more extreme position than Judaism and Christianity. In Islam, "nothing is like God," and so it rejects the Judeo-Christian idea that God made man in his own image. There are no Islamic representations of God; at most there is the word *God*, which is often beautifully represented in calligraphy. Submission to God is practiced through the five pillars—declaration of faith ("There is no deity but God and Muhammad is the Messenger of God"), ritual prayer five times a day facing Mecca, almsgiving (in the form of a tax on savings), daytime fasting during Ramadan, and the Hajj, or pilgrimage to Mecca.

Consistent with the fundamental belief in the unity of God, for Muslims, Muhammad does not have divine status in the way that Christ does for Christians. Muslims, unlike Jews, recognize Jesus Christ as an important prophet, alongside Abraham and Moses, but like Jews, they reject the idea that Christ was the incarnation of God. While Christ's message is accepted as important, Muhammad is believed to be the final prophet or messenger conveying God's will for humanity to prepare them for the final judgment day. As such, he has a unique status and requires a distinct level of love and respect. For many Muslims, it is an offense to represent Muhammad in any way. This belief can be seen in its most drastic form by the extreme reaction of some Muslims to the caricatures of Muhammad in Western publications. Whereas many Muslims revere Muhammad deeply and aim to follow his example, they do not worship him. Rather, their lives are devoted to God and to living in submission to the will of God.

The Quran is the holy book of Islam. It is an account of the revelations made to Muhammad and is therefore believed by Muslims to be the literal word of God. It describes a variety of sins and, like Judaism and Christianity, distinguishes between major and minor sins. It also distinguishes between sins against God, such as not performing one's prayers, sins against other persons, such as theft or breaking a promise, and sins against the self, such as drinking alcohol. The elaboration of sins in the Quran lies somewhere between Judaism and Christianity. Like Judaism, there are many prohibitions with respect to diet and appearance, but many more of the rules remain in effect in contemporary Islamic society. Indeed, in Islam, to a much greater extent than in Christianity and Judaism, the religious rules for behavior as outlined in the Quran are coincident with the laws of the state. In Muslim states that practice sharia law, the law is essentially an interpretation of the Quran and the Sunnah (or practice of the Prophet). In the same way, guilt in Islam is an objective state of affairs associated with transgression of religious laws.

Forgiveness plays a central role in Islamic culture. Its significance is seen right at the root of humanity's relationship with God when Adam and Eve disobeyed God in the Garden of Eden. In the Christian tradition, Adam's sin is inherited by his descendants, but in the Islamic account of the Fall, Adam repents and God forgives him, thereby resolving the first sin. Humans may retain a propensity to sin, but they are not tainted with original sin because of God's forgiveness. As a result, repentance and forgiveness have a central place in Islamic teachings, but there is no need for a savior figure like Jesus Christ.[18] Islam explicitly distinguishes between three forms of forgiveness. God can forgive people, people can forgive people, and people can forgive themselves. In Islam, it is understood that God can see into people's hearts and therefore knows when they are repentant. As a result, there is no need for a formal confession. God will forgive someone of sin if they are genuinely repentant. But forgiveness by God is not always necessary or indeed enough. Whereas one can seek God's forgiveness for sins against God, such as not abiding by the requirement for prayer or fasting, sins against persons, such as physical harm or property theft or damage, cannot be forgiven by God alone. Forgiveness must be sought from those who have been sinned against. Islam thus recognizes an explicit role for person-to-person forgiveness. It is a requirement of Islam that before undertaking *Hajj*—the pilgrimage to Mecca—Muslims must visit family, friends, and acquaintances and ask for forgiveness for any previous wrongs. It is important that such person-to-person forgiveness can even supersede the invocation of punishment by the State. Although murder normally warrants the death penalty under Islamic law, in the Quran, God allows that someone who has murdered can be spared the death penalty if the victim's kin are willing to forgive. Indeed, those who forgive in this way are promised rewards and high status in the eyes of God. This can lead to a situation where a murderer will be spared execution if the victim's kin are willing to forgive the crime.

The experience of guilt is prominent in Muslim cultures, but it appears to occur most powerfully in relation to parental authority. The family is the core social structure in Muslim culture. The Quran is explicit that honoring one's parents is a moral requirement, second only to honoring God. Loyalty to one's parents is of utmost importance. However, Islam recognizes that blind obedience by children is undesirable, particularly if a parental directive is itself sinful or unreasonable. Indeed, parents do not have the right to command obedience to their will; rather, they have an obligation to let their children develop as individuals as long as they follow God's will. The ideal family relationships involve reciprocal responsibility, whereby parents provide love and guidance that is consistent with God's will, and children should love, respect, and obey their parents. Guilt, then, emerges when these two sets of interests do not coincide, for example, when an adult child decides on a life path that the parents do not approve of.

Monotheism and Attachment to God

Guilt is prevalent in the Abrahamic religions both in an objective sense, as sin, which is the contravention of God's laws, and in the subjective sense of an emotion that the faithful experience. As we have seen, that subjective sense of guilt often arises in the context of the believer's relationship with the one true God. Research has shown that the amount of guilt that believers feel is related to the strength of their "religiosity," which essentially means the extent to which they adhere to religious beliefs and practice religious engagement.[19] There are subtle differences across the Abrahamic religions in how the relationship with God is conceived, and these differences seem to lead to some interesting differences for the experience of religious guilt. For Christians, the relationship with God most clearly resembles that between child and parent. God is "the Father." The opening line of the Lord's Prayer makes this clear: "Our Father, who art in heaven."

Christian doctrine is explicit about the similarity between God and parent, and it places God's nature at the origin of this similarity. God is powerful, omniscient, loving, merciful, punishing at times, and so on. Christianity urges parents to copy God's nature in the way they parent their children. In this way, their children will grow up to lead a good life in the eyes of God. From this religious point of view, good parenting reflects the way God is.

A psychological interpretation flips this connection around.[20] From a psychological point of view, it is children's propensity to form an attachment relationship with their parents that primes them to accept a God figure in their lives. As we have seen, attachment is the emotional bond that develops early in life to keep children safe and cared for by their parents, and children are very sensitive to threats to their attachment. The fear of separation underlies the guilt children feel in relation to their parents and the growth of conscience. The attachment bonds that are formed between children and their attachment figures persist throughout life and serve as the models for other loving relationships. Attachments are loving relationships that serve to reduce anxiety and generate a feeling of security or safety. This is exactly the emotional pattern that Christians report about their relationship to God. God is a source of infinite love, and God also protects and keeps the believer safe. God offers the emotional stability for the believer to take on the challenges that life offers. As Swedish psychologist Pehr Granqvist says, "It is not difficult to fathom how an attachment figure who is simultaneously omnipresent, omniscient, and omnipotent—all very impressive qualities that are likely to make other attachment figures green with envy—can provide the most secure of secure bases."[21] With God as super-parent, it is no surprise that Christians experience the most guilt of all believers when they fear they have threatened their relationship with God. They are in effect placed in a lifelong attachment relationship with their supernatural parent.

The idea of God the Father is most prevalent in Christian texts, including the New Testament of the Bible, but it also appears in the sacred texts of Judaism, including the Old Testament. Certainly, however, Judaism downplays the idea of God as the father of humanity, and so God is less obviously an attachment figure. Jacob Arlow, in his classic review of guilt in Judaism, puts it like this: "God is not identifiable in any way as a person; no plastic representation is permitted. In addition, there is no intermediary between God and man. Accordingly, moral judgments become personal, individual, intrapsychic responsibilities."[22] God's role in Islam is also not that of a parent. The Quran refers to God as "Lord" but not as father. God is the creator and the provider, but humans are not the children of God. These differences among the Abrahamic religions, along with the explicit imagery for God as father in Christianity, suggests that Christians may be most likely to feel a parental attachment relationship with God and most likely to feel guilt in relation to God. However, to my knowledge, there is no formal research in comparative religion that directly assesses this question.

The Role of Conscience in Religion

We have looked at the roles of both objective guilt (or sin) and the experience of guilt for believers in the Abrahamic religions, but what of conscience, the internal voice that guides us in matters of morality? All three Abrahamic religious traditions recognize the importance of conscience as a faculty of mind that allows us to follow God's laws in pursuit of a virtuous life.[23] Certainly, conscience is understood in part to be an internalized sense of fear of God's wrath for wrongdoing. This is strongly reminiscent of the Freudian idea of the superego—fear over damaging our relationship with God motivates us to follow the rules. But, the religious concept of conscience also involves a personal understanding of right and wrong.[24] It can be tricky to reconcile the idea of a personal conscience with the fact that rules for virtuous behavior are immutable, having been passed down from God. Fixed laws leave little leeway for personal choice. We can point to two principles that insert a role for personal choice. First, notwithstanding the fact that coercion has been all too common in the history of Abrahamic religious culture, it is still understood broadly that a virtuous life requires that adopting a religion is a free personal choice. The virtuous person, whether Jewish, Christian, or Muslim, is not coerced into following the rules of their religion; they adopt them freely and willingly because they care about their relationship with God.[25] They recognize that they are corruptible (or already corrupted in the case of original sin) and that following the will of God is the solution to this corruption. That is why, for example, Catholics now celebrate the sacrament of confirmation when the child is deemed old enough to make a personal commitment to the faith, and

Anabaptist denominations, descended from the Christian Reformation in the sixteenth century, postpone baptism until adulthood, when the individual can make a personal choice to be baptized. Once a person has freely decided to follow a religious path, religious teachings will nurture the internal sense of right and wrong in accordance with God's law. In this way, conscience acts as the bridge between the objective guilt or sin determined by religious laws and the subjective guilt experienced by the sinner.

Second, even within the constraints of religious dictates, there is room for a difference in opinion and personal choice regarding the right course of action. The transformative role of individual conscience is a constant throughout the evolution of the Abrahamic religions. Remember, Abraham himself reasoned with God about the morality of destroying the corrupt city of Sodom given that a small minority of its citizens were likely virtuous: "Shall not the judge of all the earth do right?"[26] The founding of Islam rested on the prophet Muhammad's personal revelation of God's will and led him to undertake a revolution and reconfiguration of the religious world of the Arabian peninsula. And Martin Luther, arguably the most important figure in the evolution of Christianity in the last five hundred years, initiated the Reformation by explicitly invoking his conscience as his guide in resisting the edicts of the Catholic Church in favor of his own interpretation of the will of God.[27] Of course, these individuals are towering figures in the history of the Abrahamic religions. Nevertheless, they show by example that authentically and fervently held personal positions on matters of morality have a critical role to play in religious practice and experience.

In everyday life, the role of conscience is more often to remind the believer of appropriate, religiously guided action. Sometimes, it can be overbearing and not particularly valuable, as I experienced that evening long ago in France. But more often, it works effectively as a guide to keep one aligned with one's religious culture. And then, every so often, one's conscience can bring about a moral conflict with one's received religion. Often, such conflict can be accommodated within the flexibility of practice that the religion offers. But sometimes, as in my own case, it can lead to an irreparable rift, and the received religion is left behind.

With this exploration of the Abrahamic religions, we have begun to examine how objective guilt and subjective guilt interact in human life and society. The Abrahamic religions all have codes of behavior that essentially define guilt in an objective sense. If a believer contravenes a religious directive, it doesn't matter whether they feel guilty for doing so; they *are* guilty of sin. Broadly speaking, sins recognize and prohibit various forms of relationship damage, where the relationship can be with God or with other persons, particularly those who are members of the family or community. But the feeling of guilt is also part of religious experience. Guilt from the fear of damaging one's relationship with God is a large part of the motivation to follow the rules. And when following the rules is tied up so intricately with family and community relationships, guilt from hurting these relationships provides an additional spur to conform. Because sin inevitably occurs, Abrahamic religious cultures recognize the need for practicing contrition and atonement by the sinner and, in return, forgiveness by those sinned against. In this way, both the objective and subjective guilt can be expunged and the relationships with God, family, and community restored.

The moral codes of the Abrahamic religions capture and share certain basic principles about how to manage one's human relationships: respecting and caring for others, honoring one's family and community, contrition and forgiveness, and so on. They differ mostly in their rules for how to honor one's relationship with God and other religious figures such as Jesus Christ and Muhammad. Increasing secularization, particularly in the West,[28] may mean that the religious beliefs and practices that honor these religious relationships are in decline. And with this decline will come a decrease in religious guilt. However, the core principles of social harmony that religions convey are more fundamental to human nature. Even as more people leave organized religion and a connection to God behind, secular modes of social organization are well-placed to step up and ensure that these principles continue to be the bedrock on which society is built and that guilt, in both its objective and subjective forms, will continue to help guide moral behavior. One critical form of organization is the law, to which we now turn.

Chapter Ten

Guilt in the Law

At about four o'clock on a freezing January night in 2018, in a peaceful residential area of Calgary, Alberta, Mount Royal University professor Janet Hamnett was awoken by what she later described as the sound of an explosion. She got out of bed and went toward the door of her bedroom, but before she could leave, she encountered the "huge presence" of Matthew Brown, the ex-captain of the Mount Royal University hockey team. Although they were both members of the same university community, they had never previously met. Brown was wielding the broken handle of a broom and making incomprehensible grunting noises. He proceeded to beat Hamnett, who raised her arms to protect her face and head and, in so doing, suffered serious damage to her hands. Hamnett was able to escape to her bathroom and lock the door, only emerging when the house had gone quiet. She made her way to the adjacent house and banged on the door, arousing her neighbors, who called the Calgary police and ambulance service. The police later found Brown lying in the bathroom of another house close by and arrested him. He was charged with multiple criminal offenses, including breaking and entering, and assault with a weapon.

At his trial, Brown admitted his responsibility, expressed remorse, and offered a heartfelt apology to Hamnett and her family. Those who observed him in court, including members of Hamnett's family, were convinced he felt enormously guilty. At the same time, he entered a plea of not guilty. His defense argued that he had committed the crimes while in a state of automatism, whereby he had no awareness of what he was doing, and so was not *criminally* responsible. That night, he had attended a party, drank a large amount of alcohol, and also took about 2.5 grams of magic mushrooms, containing the potent hallucinogen psilocybin. He had no memory of the rest of the night. The court was told that while at the party, he had stripped naked and wandered off into the night in freezing weather. The police had, indeed, found him naked and incoherent when they arrested him. Brown's defense rested on a challenge to the constitutionality of Section 33.1 of the Criminal Code of Canada, which says that reduced intentionality with respect to a criminal offense brought on by self-induced intoxication cannot be offered as a defense. Brown's counsel took the position that in his drug-induced automatism, there was not just reduced intentionality, there was no intentionality. Furthermore, Brown could not have predicted this situation based on his previous experience with such drugs. As a result, his constitutional right to have his mental state considered in the assessment of his legal responsibility was violated by the application of Section 33.1. Brown was acquitted of the charges against him, but this acquittal was reversed on appeal by the Alberta Court of Appeal. The case then made its way to the Supreme Court of Canada, which, in a controversial decision, found that Section 33.1 of the Criminal Code did, indeed, violate the Canadian Charter of Rights and Freedoms, and that, therefore, the original decision on the Brown case should be upheld. Brown was acquitted of all charges against him.

At the end of this protracted legal case, Matthew Brown was found not guilty of assault even though there was no disputing that he had beaten Janet Hamnett and left her with permanent damage to her hands. Was justice served in this case? It depends on who you talk to. Clearly, the highest court in the land believed the outcome was just. But in an interview after the initial trial, Lara Unsworth, Janet Hamnett's daughter, expressed the family's disenchantment with the outcome: "The person he is and how badly he feels has nothing to do with our disappointment; it's the actions he took and that he's not being held accountable for that, and I think they're two separate things."[1] She called for a solution, perhaps involving restorative justice, whereby some good would come out of the situation.[2]

Here, we have a perfect modern-day illustration of the difference between *feeling* guilty and *being* guilty, and of the challenges of establishing guilt under the law. When I first read about the case, I was struck by how the dissociation between feeling guilty and being guilty was the exact reverse of what I had experienced. In my own case, I was guilty under the law but, having been forgiven by those I had harmed, I did not *feel* guilty about the crime itself. Matthew Brown felt guilty for what he had done but was found not guilty of the alleged crimes under the law. As criminologist and legal scholar Howard Zehr put it: "In the legal system, offenses and questions of guilt are framed in terms much different from how the victim and the offender actually experience them."[3]

My argument throughout this book has been that guilt is connected to causing harm to social relationships. The *feeling* of guilt occurs most often when one has harmed a relationship within one's communal circle. It is a fundamental psychological mechanism for managing our social relationships in everyday life because it motivates us to resolve conflict and heal the rifts that inevitably occur periodically in these relationships. But beyond the circle of our communal relationships, the feeling of guilt starts to lose its potency. We are less likely to feel guilt in the same way with strangers. Conscience provides an important mechanism for managing social relations with people we do not know. But conscience is an individual personal experience, varying to some extent according to the guidance provided within the unique set of significant relationships that we encounter during development as well as our own moral stance on how to engage with others. To ensure uniformity in social behavior across all members of society, human cultures evolved forms of objective guilt to manage social relations among all members of larger social groups. The moral codes of religions provide one form of objective guilt. However, legal systems are the most refined approach to objective guilt yet established in human societies.

Guilt in the Law

The oldest preserved code of law is the Code of Ur-Nammu from the Sumerian civilization, dating from about 2100 BCE.* Sumer was one of the earliest agriculture-based urban civilizations of Mesopotamia, or what is now southern Iraq. It is likely no coincidence that codes of law arose as civilizations such as Sumer grew to encompass settled groups of

---

* Although no preserved code of law has been found to date, it is generally agreed that ancient Egypt operated with a code of law at least a thousand years earlier than the Code of Ur-Nammu. Indeed, basic laws were likely in operation in Egypt in the predynastic period from 6000 BCE.

people numbering many thousands, well beyond the group sizes characteristic of earlier hunter-gatherer, nomadic herder, and primitive horticulturist societies. In such civilizations, the prospects for interacting with people outside of one's communal group increased considerably. The code of law supplemented more natural emotional mechanisms, such as the feeling of guilt, that only work well for managing social behavior between individuals within smaller groups.

The Code of Ur-Nammu was recorded on terra cotta tablets and is only partially preserved. Nevertheless, the structure is clear and involves a series of statements identifying a punishment or form of restitution for committing a particular crime. For example:

- If a man commits murder, that man must be killed.

- If a man knocks out a tooth of another man, he shall pay two shekels of silver.

- If a man commits a robbery, he will be killed.

- If a man divorces his first-time wife, he shall pay her one mina of silver.

- If a man appeared as a witness, and was shown to be a perjurer, he must pay fifteen shekels of silver.

As these examples illustrate, of the thirty-two statements that have survived, the majority deal with acts causing physical harm to another, crimes involving property (including slaves), and practices particular to family relations. Interestingly, as the last example above illustrates, there are also statements that regulate the management of the legal system itself. If a legal system is to work, then its operation must be protected. So, as with modern legal systems, respect for the process of law is critical.

From these relatively simple beginnings, codes of law became firmly established and spread rapidly. In the English-speaking world, the dominant legal tradition is known as "common law" and traces its origin to the system of law established after the Norman conquest of

The Power of Guilt

England in the eleventh century.* In common law, there is a high-level distinction between criminal law, which covers offenses that are wrong with respect to society as a whole, and civil law, which covers disputes between private individuals or organizations, including businesses. A key difference between criminal and civil law is in how they conceive of the party that is wronged. In criminal law, offenses are deemed to be against the state or society as a whole, not against any individual who may be the victim of the offense. Generally, the concept of guilt is meaningful only in the context of criminal law. Guilt is assigned when it can be shown to the satisfaction of a court of law that the accused did, indeed, commit the crime. In contrast, in civil cases, one party makes a legal claim against another and the law works to provide a resolution of the dispute, by determining liability, not guilt. The legal system provides the framework for the resolution of the civil suit, including the court system, within which the case will be tried and resolved, but the state does not act as a party in the dispute. The court determines the remedy, often in the form of financial damages paid by one party to the other. There is no need to assign guilt.*

Because crimes are offenses against the state, it is the state or the relevant jurisdiction that brings the case against the accused to court,

---

* In the modern world, there are two main secular strands of jurisprudence. Alongside common law of the English-speaking world, there is the tradition of civil law, which is heir to the rationalization of legal codes achieved during the tenure of the Roman emperor Justinian I during the sixth century CE and was ultimately adopted in most continental European countries during the medieval period. Civil law takes a strong approach to codification of the law, with an extensive code specifying which acts are subject to prosecution, how to establish that an action is against the law, and what punishment is appropriate. In the present day, most countries of continental Europe, the countries that were colonized by them, including those in Central and South America and much of Africa, as well as other nations looking to adopt a codified legal tradition now follow civil law. Alongside the two main secular legal traditions, there are other codes of law rooted in religion. The most widely used is sharia law, which is based on the legal interpretation of the Islamic holy works—the Quran and Sunnah—and which plays a prominent role in the Islamic world.
* Although it is not typically framed in this way, I find it helpful to think of the difference between criminal and civil law in terms of the difference between communal and exchange relationships, which we reviewed in Chapter 5. Civil law manages relationships in terms of fairness in the exchange of benefits, whereas criminal law manages relationships where there is a fundamental breakdown in caring.

not the victim. So, when Matthew Brown was charged with assault with a weapon after beating Janet Hamnett, he was accused of a crime against the state, not against Hamnett herself, and the case was brought by the prosecutor on behalf of the state. It may seem counterintuitive, but in this case, from a legal point of view, Hamnett could serve only as a witness to the alleged crime. This is why this Canadian case is recorded as *R. v. Brown*—the R stands for *Rex* (King) or *Regina* (Queen), who, as is the case in the UK, represents the state in Canada. In the US, which is a republic, cases are recorded with "The People" as the prosecutor.

Why are criminal offenses deemed to be against the state? There are two main reasons; one relates to the nature of crime and the other to the consequences that can be imposed. First, crimes are transgressions that are deemed to be wrong in our society, no matter who the victim is. For example, murder is a crime irrespective of who is murdered. This is a critically important feature of the law, as it strives to protect all citizens and support fundamental human rights for all. Criminal law removes personal relationships almost entirely from the consideration of guilt, and as a result, the subjective experience of guilt is replaced by objective guilt under the law. Second, and more practically, crimes are transgressions that activate various potential consequences that only the state can impose, such as incarceration, monetary fines, or even death, as is still the case in some jurisdictions.

To see how the concept of guilt works in the legal system, we can look at three aspects of the system. First, there are the laws themselves, which provide the directives to members of society on how to act or how not to act. Second, there are the legal processes that enable the determination of whether someone is guilty of breaking a law. Third, there is the legal judgment on how to resolve the guilt.

Kinds of Crimes

Legal systems are built around a set of laws that guide human behavior by issuing prohibitions on certain kinds of behavior. Laws have their origins in moral or religious codes such as the Ten Commandments, but they have evolved over time with the increasing complexity of society. In common law jurisdictions such as the UK, Canada, and the US, laws include both prior court rulings (or what is known as case law) and statutes, which are pieces of legislation enacted by a governing body, such as Parliament in Canada and the UK, or Congress in the US. The evolution through history of the range of offenses deemed to be criminal has largely been an organic process of growth and refinement as legal cases and legislative acts add to, subtract from, or modify the catalogue of crimes and how they should be managed. Given the organic evolution of the law, legal authorities have struggled to organize recognized crimes into a code reflecting a taxonomy based on systematic principles.[4] It is notable that the UK, the birthplace of the common law system of jurisprudence, has not managed to produce a comprehensive criminal code despite repeated calls for one and the establishment of a law commission to formulate one well over thirty years ago. Both the US and Canada do have criminal codes. The US has a complex system of state and federal criminal codes operating side by side.[5] Criminal law is largely the jurisdiction of the individual states. As a result, there is a large variety of state-specific criminal codes recognizing, and providing guidance on the prosecution of, different kinds of crimes. An action that is illegal in one state may not be in another. In addition, in 1948, the US federal government enacted Title 18 to recognize a range of criminal offenses, some of which pertain to national responsibilities. Title 18 has approximately 120 chapters describing many kinds of crime. It is perhaps telling that these chapters are ordered alphabetically rather than in reference to any meaningful taxonomy of criminal offense. Canada has a single national criminal code, first established in 1892, that outlines the range of criminal offenses and the legal processes for determining guilt under the law.[6] But this code too looks more like a laundry list of crimes than an organized model for how the various offenses fit together.

Is there a way to make sense of the enormous range and variety of crimes that exist in modern legal codes? I have argued throughout this book that guilt serves to manage our social relationships. Criminal guilt carries out this function for people who don't necessarily know each other but who are all part of a larger community—their society. All criminal offenses identify prohibited actions that cause some form of harm to other people, but those harmed can range from individual persons to groups of people to society as a whole. If we stand back and look at bodies of criminal law through a lens that shows how the criminalization of different kinds of actions serves to manage our relationships within society, then we can see that in essentially all cases, some form of relationship has been harmed, from the particular to the more abstract. I am most familiar with the Canadian legal system, so let me take a bit of a deeper dive into the Criminal Code of Canada, as an example of a contemporary criminal code, to see how the types of crimes it identifies fit this model.

The Criminal Code of Canada was first drafted in 1892 and has served as the core legal code for crimes in Canada ever since.* Over time, many amendments have occurred. The Criminal Code now includes the following main sections that lay out the categories of criminal offenses:[7]

> Part II—Offences Against Public Order
>
> Part III—Firearms and Other Weapons
>
> Part IV—Offences Against the Administration of Law and Justice
>
> Part V—Sexual Offences, Public Morals and Disorderly Conduct
>
> Part VI—Invasion of Privacy
>
> Part VII—Disorderly Houses, Gaming and Betting
>
> Part VIII—Offences Against the Person and Reputation
>
> Part VIII.1—Offences Relating to Conveyances
>
> Part IX—Offences Against Rights of Property
>
> Part X—Fraudulent Transactions Relating to Contracts and Trade
>
> Part XI—Wilful and Forbidden Acts in Respect of Certain Property

---

* The Criminal Code is not the only document relevant to criminal law in Canada. It is subservient to the Charter of Rights and Freedoms, which provides for the basic human rights that all citizens enjoy, such as the right to free expression, and various legal and democratic rights. It is also supplemented by many topic-specific acts that govern particular areas such as occupational health and safety, food and drug regulation, and income tax.

Part XII—Offences Relating to Currency

At the heart of the system are crimes that directly cause harm to another individual. These are the crimes that most clearly target a particular other person or persons, and they are fundamental to all criminal codes dating back to the Code of Ur-Nammu. Such crimes may involve physical harm, or threats of physical harm, including assault, sexual violence, or murder. They may also involve harm to the other person through appropriating or damaging their property (Part XI). Examples here would be theft of items or money, or intrusion into the other's personal spaces—breaking and entering and trespass (Part IX). Crimes against an individual also include offenses that violate a person's human rights, such as the right to privacy (Part VI). Finally, there are also crimes that reflect the society's determination of what are appropriate relations between individuals. Sexual relations have been a particular focus over time with laws governing who can have sexual relations with whom. The criminality of such relations has changed considerably over time as society's respect for the authority of mutual consent has increased. For example, homosexual activity was criminal in Canada until 1969, but was incrementally decriminalized in the following decades out of respect for the individual rights of consenting adults. As the justice minister, and future prime minister of Canada, Pierre Trudeau, said at the time the changes were introduced, "There's no place for the state in the bedrooms of the nation."[8]

But beyond crimes against a particular individual, there are crimes that cause harm to a broader group of people. If I drive under the influence of drugs or alcohol, I endanger the lives of everyone else who may be on or near the road at the time. My criminal activity does not target any particular person, but I am a potential threat to many other people. Other examples of behavior deemed of potential harm to many people include the distribution of pornography and disturbing the peace or being a public nuisance. Similarly, causing damage to public property, such as vandalism or arson to community buildings like churches or schools (Part IX), impact multiple people. The Code also articulates offenses relating to certain tools, such as firearms (Part III) and vehicles (Part VIII.1), that the society has determined need to be regulated or licensed to restrict the potential for causing broad harm. Finally, there is the category of hate crime that attempts to ensure that certain identifiable groups of people, based on race, ethnicity, gender, sexual orientation, or other protected characteristics, cannot be the target of propaganda or incitement to hatred (Part VIII).

And then, at the highest level of abstractness, are crimes against society as a whole. The Criminal Code of Canada groups many of these kinds of crimes under Part II—Offences Against Public Order. Perhaps the clearest example of crimes against society are treason—the perpetration of an act to undermine the government of the country—and sedition—the incitement of acts to undermine the government (Part II). Terrorism is also included in this section. Various forms of corruption, such as election tampering or bribery of government officials, prevent the state from working fairly and effectively for all citizens. Undermining the stability of the monetary system, including tax evasion and offenses relating to currency, such as counterfeiting, may also be considered crimes against society as a whole.

Finally, as a special category of crimes against society, are crimes that undermine the operation of the legal system itself. Perjury or lying under oath compromises the ability of the justice system to operate effectively. If an offender has been convicted of a crime, then failure to complete their sentence (for example, by escaping from prison) constitutes an additional crime. In the Canadian Criminal Code, such crimes fall under Part IV—Offences Against the Administration of Law and Justice.

In summary, the Criminal Code of Canada, like those of other jurisdictions, covers a very broad range of crimes from those that cause physical harm to a single person all the way through to crimes that damage the structure and operation of the society itself. The overriding principle, however, is that despite their very different natures, all crimes cause harm or damage to the relationships between people whether as individuals, collectives, or society as a whole.* All these kinds of crime are handled within the same legal structure—all are subject to similar processes to decide on whether the accused person is guilty, and all are subject to a limited set of consequences that can be imposed when the accused person is found guilty.

---

* We can contrast secular legal codes with religious codes, in which, as we saw in the last chapter, some of the sins concern the relationship with God.

The Power of Guilt

How Is Guilt Decided in Law?

In a sense, determining guilt under the law is very simple. If you break a law, then it is a fact that you are guilty. This is the essence of objective guilt and sets it apart from the forms of subjective guilt that we reviewed earlier in the book. Subjective guilt arises when we are concerned about possible damage to our relationships; it necessarily depends on how we feel about that relationship. But the law decides for us when we have harmed a relationship; how we feel about the relationship is irrelevant. The complication for objective guilt is in how to establish whether someone has, indeed, broken a law. Establishing guilt requires the collection and presentation of evidence as well as a party to assess the validity of that evidence. In Western legal traditions, evidence is presented in an adversarial format by the prosecution acting for the state and by the defense acting for the accused, or defendant. After all the evidence has been presented at trial, the court decides on the guilt of the defendant. The decision is made either by a presiding judge or panel of judges or by a jury, a group of citizens chosen to be able to deliver an impartial decision.

Standards for establishing guilt have varied greatly over time and across cultures. Currently, the general standard is to establish guilt beyond reasonable doubt, which essentially means that any rational person would judge the evidence to prove the defendant's guilt with very close to complete certainty. Whether or not the defendant feels guilt is irrelevant. The only issue is whether the evidence allows a firm conclusion that the defendant committed the crime. However, there is a role for a defendant *expressing* guilt. The defendant has a choice to plead either guilty or not guilty. Pleading guilty is a shortcut to establishing guilt under the law. When a defendant confesses their guilt and this confession is admitted into evidence, the burden of establishing proof beyond reasonable doubt is lifted, a trial becomes unnecessary, and the process can move immediately to sentencing. In the case of my own youthful crime, I chose to plead guilty because it was obvious that I had broken the law—I was found in the front seat of a vehicle that had been taken without the owner's permission. This shortcut relieves the prosecution of most of its effort, and so there is considerable motivation for prosecutors to try to extract a confession from criminal suspects. This is why the right to remain silent is recognized in the common law systems of Canada and the UK, and why the Constitution of the US includes the fifth amendment, which explicitly allows defendants to opt not to incriminate themselves. If the defendant pleads not guilty, the burden of proof of guilt falls to the prosecutor. The prosecution must present a compelling case to the court that the defendant is guilty beyond reasonable doubt. The defendant, through their counsel, will aim to introduce enough ambiguity about the evidence into the proceedings to prevent the court from finding them guilty beyond reasonable doubt.

The basic requirement for finding a defendant guilty is the demonstration that the defendant is to blame for, or at fault for, the harm that was caused. Thinking back to Matthew Brown's case, the court was asked to judge whether Matthew Brown was to blame for the harm he caused to Janet Hamnett. For most crimes, there are two key elements that must be proven to assign blame. First, it must be shown that the defendant participated in the illegal act—either they carried out the act themselves or they were an accomplice to someone else who carried out the act. This is called *actus reus*, or "guilty act." For the most part, establishing *actus reus* involves proving physical aspects of the crime. For example, can the defendant be placed at the scene of the crime? In Matthew Brown's case, there was no doubt that he caused the harm to Janet Hamnett. She testified that Brown was her assailant, and he was found by police close by in the condition that she described.

Second, there is a requirement that the defendant is blameworthy in a mental or psychological sense. This is called the *mens rea*, or "guilty mind."* The *mens rea* component ensures that causing harm without meaning to do so is not blameworthy. Matthew Brown's acquittal occurred because the court was convinced that as a result of ingesting the magic mushrooms, he had no awareness of what he was doing and so could not have meant to do it.*

---

* There are a few exceptions where *mens rea* is not required. These are called strict liability offenses, where merely carrying out the act entails guilt under the law. Statutory rape is one such offense.
* Strictly speaking, Matthew Brown's conviction failed on *actus reus* grounds, because for *actus reus* to be established, the action must be voluntary. However, voluntary action is also a precondition for intention—you cannot intend to do something unless you are aware of being able to do it, and so *mens rea* was also not established in Brown's case.

To be clear, establishing *mens rea* does not require that the defendant *knows* the act is illegal or that the defendant *feels* guilty. It only means that the defendant carried out the action with an understanding, at least to some extent, of its harmful consequences. If the defendant acted while knowing the harmful consequences, then they may be considered blameworthy whether or not they knew that the action was illegal.[9] And the feeling of guilt is irrelevant to establishing the facts of guilt under the law. This is why, as we saw in Chapter 4, psychopaths are very commonly represented in the prison population. Psychopaths who commit crimes know the consequences even though they lack the emotional experience of guilt to inhibit themselves from committing the offenses.

This mention of criminal psychopaths, who may be dispositionally inclined to commit crime, should remind us that in any particular criminal case, blameworthiness is in reference to the crime that was committed. Either the defendant is guilty or not guilty of the crime that is under investigation. It is not a finding about the character or disposition of the accused. Even though we might believe that some people are just bad, according to the law, it is actions that are bad, not people. Certainly, repeat offenders are treated differently when it comes to the repercussions of committing a crime. However, strictly speaking, this is a result of the accumulation of offenses and the inferred likelihood of a future offense, not because the offender has a criminal character. How then, are criminal acts treated by the legal system?

The Resolution of Guilt

The third aspect of the legal system is the resolution of the offender's guilt. We have seen that everyday subjective guilt is resolved when the relationship between the parties has been restored. When one person has harmed another whom they care about, the guilt they feel is what moves them to try to heal the relationship, but it generally requires forgiveness by the harmed party for this healing to occur. Forgiveness by the one harmed is the complement to the guilt that the offender feels. In criminal law, the justice system decides on guilt and then determines the consequences of that guilt. Resolution of the guilt is supposed to be achieved by the offender completing a sentence. But, as we shall see, too often, completing a sentence does not restore the offender's relationship with society, because in the justice system, true forgiveness is hard to come by.

In the traditional approach to criminal justice, once a defendant has been found guilty, the judge must decide on the sentence. At this point, the offender, and if appropriate, those directly affected by the crime, may speak to the impact of the crime. Offenders may take the opportunity to express their remorse. Where there are individual victims harmed by the offender's crime, they may provide a victim-impact statement. Having heard from all parties, the judge will impose a sentence designed to achieve one or more of four broad goals, which we can call "punishment," "rehabilitation," "protection,"* and "restitution." The first two are more focused on the offender, while the latter two are more focused on the victim.

It is fair to say that throughout history, punishment has dominated sentencing for criminal offenses. Punishment has two main aims: retribution and deterrence. Retribution is backward-looking and is essentially motivated by a form of justice—the harm wreaked by the offender should result in appropriate harm to the offender. The simple approach to retribution whereby the perpetrator suffers the same harm as that which they inflicted on the victim—"an eye for an eye"—has largely been consigned to history. However, it is still the case that the severity of the punishment will match the severity of the crime. Murder is punished more severely than manslaughter, which is punished more severely than assault. Deterrence is forward-looking in that the punishment is also presumed to discourage the offender (and other potential offenders) from committing the same or similar crime again in the future. If deterrence of this kind is to work, then the personal consequences of punishment for the offender must be aversive enough to overcome whatever benefit the offender may gain from committing the crime. At the same time, punishment should not be too severe—a balance between punishment of the offender and respect for their human rights must be achieved.

---

* What I am calling "protection" is sometimes called "incapacitance" in legal discussion.

Rehabilitation is a more constructive approach to deterrence. On the assumption that having done so once, offenders may be naturally inclined to reoffend given the chance, sentencing may include elements designed to lead offenders away from crime. Depending on the particular crime and the circumstances of the offender, rehabilitation may include programs such as drug rehab, anger management, or work skills training.

Laws exist to protect citizens and society in general from the harmful behavior of others. Everyone living in a society should be afforded protection from criminal behavior. When bad actors break the law, then action must be taken to protect those who may be at risk and the social order more generally. In some cases, the protection will require that the offenders are separated from the public. Inevitably, this removal from society requires some degree of limitation on their freedom and a penal system to accommodate offenders.

Finally, because crimes cause harm to others, it is reasonable for criminals to pay a cost to make good that harm where possible. Sentences often include a component whereby the offender is required to pay a fine or contribute some other form of payback.

If these are the reasons for sentences, then what forms do sentences take? Although, as we have seen, there is an enormous variety in types of crime, judges have a very limited variety of sentences that they can impose in response to a guilty verdict. Physical punishment was common historically, but it is now relatively rare worldwide and almost nonexistent in Western jurisdictions practicing civil or common law. Capital punishment still exists as a punishment in a minority of countries. But in their most recent global report, Amnesty International show a continuing decline in recorded executions, with only eighteen nations reporting any executions.[10] The US is the only Western nation where capital punishment is still legal, and slowly, more and more states are abolishing it. Needless to say, capital punishment, while it clearly achieves the goals of retribution, deterrence, and protection, completely prevents the possibility of an offender's crime being forgiven.

Generally, in the Western world, there are two broad categories of sentence: imposing limits on the offender's freedom and requiring the offender to provide compensation. In both cases, the sentence needs to be tailored to the crime and gauged to provide an appropriate deterrent to future criminal activity. In most jurisdictions, judges are provided guidance in law as to what sentences can be imposed for which crimes.

Limits on the offender's ability to live their life with their usual freedom are enabled by sentencing the offender to probation or jail time. These sentences serve primarily as punishment for the offender and protection for society. Ideally, they will also build in some elements of rehabilitation.

Probation is more often used as a sentence for first-time offenders or for minor crimes. It allows the offender to continue to live in the community, but certain restrictions are imposed on their day-to-day life, such as a curfew, limits on travel, or the requirement to check in regularly with a probation officer. In addition, the judge may order the offender to participate in a rehabilitation program, such as anger management or drug treatment. Failure to comply with the conditions of the probation can lead to the imposition of a prison sentence.

Jail time can range from periods as short as a few months to life imprisonment and essentially isolates the offender from all normal aspects of everyday life. Prisoners are removed from their homes, family, and friends. They cannot work and they cannot participate in their usual hobbies or pastimes. Offenders are sent to penal settings with different levels of security depending on the seriousness of their crime. These penal settings differ considerably in the activities they provide for prisoners. Penal systems often build in rehabilitation programs so that prisoners can take part in a range of programs, which are generally designed to reduce their future interest in criminal activity. Whether certain modern penal systems, such as the prison-industrial complex in the US, are faithful to this purpose is an issue of considerable debate.

When I served my prison sentence, I spent time in two quite different penal settings. I was initially sent to a high-security prison, where I was locked in a bare cell with one other prisoner for the whole day and night except for bathroom breaks and one hour of exercise. I was then transferred to a minimum-security "open" prison. There, I slept in a dormitory, where I could interact with a range of other inmates. I worked in the prison laundry, and in my free time, I walked the prison grounds at my leisure, played cards or dominos with other prisoners, or read books that I was allowed to receive from the outside. I could also participate in a range of educational programs and took the opportunity to join an introductory class in German. The open prison provided considerable limits on my freedom, but it was a completely different experience compared to the high-security prison. In open prison, I was also struck by the variety of inmates' crimes. There were no violent criminals—they were not eligible for open prison—but I was surrounded by petty burglars, white collar embezzlers, serial drunk drivers, drug dealers. I could not help but wonder whether society was well served by treating such an array of characters in the same way.

When I reflect on how I felt in the two settings where I spent my jail time, I think I gained some insight into the ways in which incarceration both punishes and deters criminals. Having one's liberty removed by being sent to prison is supposed to be punishment in itself. But in the high-security prison, the lack of freedom to engage in almost any meaningful activity made me feel as if I was being punished every day I was there. In the open prison, I accepted that I had been punished by being sent there, but once there, I was able to participate in a facsimile of society, engage in different activities, interact with different people, and build a degree of self-respect within the boundaries of my confinement. The difference between these two forms of incarceration brought home to me the different purposes that prison sentences for criminal convictions can serve. For someone like me, whose crime was the result of a momentary act of recklessness, open prison provided more than enough punishment to deter me from future criminal activity. Indeed, I think the subjective guilt I felt in the aftermath of the accident served as a greater deterrent than being found guilty under the law. But I observed others in the prison who took advantage of the flexibility and lack of oversight to operate successful illegal activities, such as businesses trading smuggled drugs and alcohol. I doubt open prison made much of an impact on their future criminal careers.

Compensation involves requiring the offender to repay in some way the debt to society that they have incurred through their criminal behavior. The simplest form of compensation in effect monetizes the impact of a crime. A fine is levied in accordance with the harm that has been caused. As we saw earlier, all crimes are technically against the state, and therefore monetary fines for criminal offenses are usually paid to the state. However, where the crime has caused financial hardship to a victim, judges may require offenders to pay damages to cover the costs incurred by the individuals who have been directly harmed by the offenders' actions. Judges may also impose a sentence involving some form of community service as restitution. Community service involves the offender doing unpaid work in the community. It may be relatively menial, like clearing litter from public spaces, or it may require offenders to donate their time to talk to community groups about the offense they committed and its impact on their lives.

Does Criminal Justice Ever Resolve Guilt?

By completing a sentence, a person convicted of a crime is supposed to have paid their debt to society, and their guilt has been dealt with. But has it really? As we have seen, traditional forms of sentence tend to focus on the management of the offender or on the needs of the public. These sentences rarely focus on how to restore the relationship between offender and society. If the relationship is to be restored, then forgiveness of the offender by the state is an important part of this healing. Are those who serve sentences for criminal offenses ever genuinely forgiven? Unfortunately, the legal system is set up to make complete forgiveness of offenders a relative rarity. And, if offenders are never truly forgiven by the state, then the relationship between offender and society may remain broken.

One of the most destructive practices for forgiveness is the maintenance of criminal records. All jurisdictions maintain records of anyone who has been convicted of a crime. A criminal offense ensures a permanent stain on offenders' records as far as the criminal justice system is concerned. Although the justice system is supposed to identify and manage guilty behavior, the criminal record means that criminal guilt becomes a property of the offender. The crime is part of the person's identity as far as the law is concerned, and it can follow them for life. A person found guilty of break and enter becomes a burglar. A person who has spent time in prison becomes an ex-con. The criminal record tells society not to fully trust its holder, and by the same token, it tells its holder that society does not fully trust them.

Keeping criminal records is, of course, entirely understandable. If a suspect in a break-and-enter crime is found to have a similar previous conviction, then that is an important piece of evidence in the investigation of the crime. And it also suggests that the consequences for the crime should be more severe. Furthermore, protection of the public may require ongoing restrictions of convicted offenders who may be prone to reoffend. As a parent, I would certainly want convicted pedophiles to be prevented from interacting with my child. However, the use of criminal records can go far beyond their reasonable use within the legal system. If I had committed my crime today, it is possible that my chosen career as a developmental psychologist would have been denied me. These days, all my students who want to work with children in a research setting are required to undergo a criminal record check and cannot be involved in testing children if the check does not come up clean. If such standards had been in effect when I was a student, they might have effectively prevented me from doing my PhD and going on to a career as a professor and researcher. Potential employers, landlords, and financial institutions all may make use of criminal record checks. As a result, a citizen with a criminal record may be denied work, housing, and financial support.

These effects can occur in a systematic manner within society with devastating consequences. In her classic book, *The New Jim Crow*, Michelle Alexander shows how the use of criminal records has helped to create a self-perpetuating cycle of criminality for many Black Americans.[11] One relatively minor drug conviction, for which the "war on drugs" mandated prison sentences, can set in motion a cascade of effects that make it essentially impossible for the person to clamber back onto the ladder of success after serving their sentence. After release from prison, the ex-convict's first task may be to find housing, but they have now become ineligible for public housing and must declare their criminal record if asked by private landlords. The result is that many ex-convicts become homeless. Then the ex-convict must try to find a job, but now encounters employers who require both a permanent address and a criminal record check for employment. The likelihood of being hired for almost any job plummets with a criminal record, particularly for Black men. Without a means of supporting oneself, one would hope that welfare might kick in, but in many states in the US, individuals with drug-related convictions are also ineligible for welfare. Without suitable housing, meaningful work, and government support, ex-convicts are clearly sent a message that they are not wanted and will never be considered to have paid their debt to society. As Michelle Alexander demonstrates, the justice system pursuant to the war on drugs is set up to *deny* forgiveness to those convicted of crimes. Little wonder, then, that with such limited other options, they often fall back into a life of criminal behavior.

Given the stigma and repercussions associated with a criminal record, the best outcome for a convicted offender is a pardon. The meaning of *pardon* varies greatly across jurisdictions, but in many, including Canada and the US, it amounts to forgiveness for the crime of which the person was convicted. With a pardon, the criminal record of the offender may be sealed so that it cannot be accessed through request by the police or any other party, or it may be expunged, whereby it is completely destroyed. Unfortunately, the use of pardons is quite limited, applying mainly to wrongful convictions and convictions now considered to be unjust based on the evolution of the law, such as convictions in Canada prior to 1969 for homosexual acts. Under these conditions, the person who was convicted of a crime is considered never to have committed a crime. In Canada, efforts to recognize the discrimination that convicted offenders face upon release have been partially addressed by a program that has replaced the pardon, called "record suspension," whereby criminal record checks do not reveal that the person committed a crime. Most people convicted of a crime can apply for record suspension after certain conditions have been met, including that the person has completed all aspects of their sentence, that a waiting period of at least five years (for minor offenses) or up to ten years (for major crimes) has passed, and that the person has demonstrated good behavior during that period. Record suspension is not available to those convicted of sexual crimes against minors and those with three or more serious convictions. Only 4 percent of those with successful record suspension have it withdrawn subsequently because of a further crime, which shows that the vast majority never commit another crime and deserve their forgiveness.[12] Nevertheless, the proportion of those who are eligible to apply who go through the process remains a minority, meaning that most people convicted of a crime never receive forgiveness.

Restoring the Relationship between Offender and Society

In 1974, a landmark criminal case occurred in Elmira, Ontario, Canada.[13] There was nothing particularly remarkable about the crime itself. Two youths got drunk and went on a rampage, slashing tires, smashing windows, and damaging fences in their community. They were charged with twenty-two counts of willful damage to property. The probation officer assigned to the case, Mark Yantzi, suggested in his report for the court that "there could be some therapeutic value in having the offenders meet their victims." The presiding judge picked up on the idea, and even though there was no legal precedent for such an approach, he followed through on the suggestion. Along with a fine and a requirement to pay restitution to the victims, the judge directed the offenders to meet and apologize to the community members whose property they had destroyed. The offenders, who had been on a path to jail and a potential lifetime of criminality, were profoundly changed by the experience. Their criminal guilt became supplemented by an emotional experience of guilt as they came face to face with the members of their community whom they hurt. One of them, Russ Kelly, who had lost both his parents as a child and was, as a teenager, already directionless and addicted to drugs and alcohol, became so involved in community work that he was recognized twenty-five years later with a lifetime community service award by the Toronto Police. So it was that the application of community justice, which is now more commonly known as "restorative justice," to criminal cases was introduced into the criminal justice system.

The restorative justice approach casts offenders and victims as parties in a web of relationships. As Howard Zehr, a criminologist and legal scholar, says in his book *Changing Lenses*, which introduced the restorative justice approach to a larger audience, "[C]rime is a violation of people and relationships. It creates obligations to make things right. Justice involves the victim, the offender, and the community in a search for solutions which promote repair, reconciliation, and reassurance."[14] Even if the offender and victim have no relationship prior to the crime, the crime itself creates a relationship, one in which the offender has harmed the victim. Offenders and victims are also in other relationships that may be affected by the crime. Maybe the offender has their own family that would be impacted by their incarceration. As we have seen, many crimes don't just affect a particular other person; they may impact many, so that a whole community may be harmed. My own experience with crime just five years after the Elmira case was consistent with this idea. In stealing the car and playing my part in the death of a fellow student, I had harmed not only the students who had been the victims of the accident, but their families and friends, my own family and friends, and the whole university community. The focus on the web of relationships affected by the crime moves the consideration of the resolution of guilt beyond punishment of the offender and compensation of the immediate victims to include the healing of all those relationships.

The principles of the restorative approach are not new. They are at the heart of many smaller communities' natural approaches to justice. Introducing restorative justice approaches into criminal law has resonated strongly with Indigenous communities. These approaches have been embraced in North America, where traditional Indigenous approaches to community justice have influenced how restorative justice is practiced in the legal system. Drawing on Māori customs, restorative justice has now become standard practice for youth crime in New Zealand. The growth in a restorative justice approach to the resolution of guilt in the criminal justice system is an explicit recognition that the outcomes of the legal process may be enhanced through engaging offender, victims, and their communities together in a consideration of how best to resolve the offender's guilt.

As a general approach, restorative justice brings offenders, victims, and other affected community members together in a dialogue that is supported by facilitators. An essential part of any resolution is to explore what the victims and their community need from the justice system and from the offenders to find peace. At the same time, offenders are asked to reflect on the harm they have caused to the victims and to the community. This reflection encourages them to focus on the impact of their crime and to take responsibility for it. One of the great benefits of the restorative approach is that the resolution of criminal offenses can be tailored in a more refined way to the particular circumstances of offenders and victims. In addition, offenders and victims are offered an opportunity to see each other as people whose actions have reasons, which can spark empathy for each other. Seeing each other in this way yields the possibility for genuine remorse, empathy, and forgiveness.

Where the traditional legal approach to justice is focused on objective guilt, the relational basis of the restorative approach brings subjective and objective guilt together in the criminal justice system.[15] Objective, legal guilt still applies and must be demonstrated, but the approach encourages offenders to experience their crimes in a way that stimulates the feeling of guilt also.

I do not mean to give the impression that restorative justice can replace the traditional criminal justice system. Sometimes, victims seek only retribution, so they reject participation in restorative justice practices with those who harmed them. Sometimes, criminals feel no remorse or need to change and would do the same thing given the opportunity, so they too reject participation in restorative justice. The idea of criminal guilt and more punitive methods of response remain essential for managing such cases. But where there is the possibility that recruiting subjective guilt, with its combination of remorse and empathy, to aid in the management of crime and achieve longer lasting change, restorative justice provides an important alternative to an exclusive focus on objective guilt determined by criminal justice.

I began this chapter with *R. v. Brown*, an important case in recent Canadian law. Matthew Brown was found not guilty of assaulting Janet Hamnett, even though it was indisputable that he had beaten her and even though he felt guilt and remorse for doing so. Such cases are important in the criminal justice system for working through the complications of what it means to be guilty under the law. *R. v. Brown* led directly to the rewriting of a section of the Criminal Code of Canada. Nevertheless, such cases can leave one dissatisfied with the way the law may work for individual cases. Certainly, Janet Hamnett and her family were displeased with the outcome. Incorporating a restorative approach, whereby all parties can engage together to resolve the outcomes of an offense to their mutual satisfaction, offers hope for victims, offenders, their communities, and society more generally to repair the harm that crime wreaks.

Just as the feeling of guilt serves to manage our important communal relationships, legal systems and the concept of criminal guilt are designed to achieve the same outcomes for society at large. Legal processes mimic the psychology of guilt. The existence of laws alerts us to when someone has damaged relationships within society, and the legal system provides the means to resolve the guilt through prosecution and the fulfillment of a sentence. The legal system also serves a similar function to conscience—it acts as a guide for acceptable behavior and discourages actions that are harmful to relationships within society.

Guilt, whether as feeling or fact, can only truly be relieved by forgiveness. That is why we need to recognize that when criminal guilt has occurred, the possibility of forgiveness should always be considered. Punishment for breaking the law is important and necessary for reasons of justice and deterrence. But alone, punishment is not sufficient. In an ideal world, the relationship between the transgressor and the harmed, whether individual victims or the state, would be rebuilt. The consequences of criminal guilt would be designed with reconciliation between offender and society in mind. Of course, society may determine that in certain cases of criminal guilt, the relationship is too broken to be recovered and the risk for reoffense is too great. An emphasis on the protection of society, and therefore ongoing offender punishment, will be warranted in those cases. But, equally, in those cases, one might suggest that guilt has failed in its purpose of relationship repair.

Chapter Eleven

Collective Guilt

It was a late fall evening and I was sitting in the car waiting. The temperature was dropping fast, so I was guiltily keeping the motor running and turned up the car heater. I had driven Shannon to the condo she rents out to visiting academics and professionals. She was checking the washer/dryer because her current tenant was having a problem with it. A few minutes later, she came out of the condo and got in the car. I could see immediately that something was wrong. She was visibly upset, and I asked her what had happened.

"Romesh just told me that he has been racially abused."

Romesh was a new Indian junior professor, hired at my university as part of an affirmative action program to increase the number of racially visible faculty members. He had only arrived a few weeks ago and was staying at Shannon's condo while he looked for his own place.

"I was just asking him how things were going, and he said, 'Fine, except for the people.' He told me he was walking down Spring Garden Road to do some shopping and someone said to him, 'Go back to where you came from. You don't belong here.' I said, 'What a jerk,' and he immediately said, 'It wasn't just once—I've been told that a number of times.' I was completely taken aback and embarrassed. I felt so guilty that Nova Scotians would do that. I just said how sorry I was that he had been treated like that."

"But you don't have anything to be guilty about it—you didn't do anything wrong," I said.

"I know, but these are my people," she responded.

When I think back to this incident (which happened before I started working on this book), I realize how, at the time, I completely missed the essence of what had happened in this exchange between Shannon and Romesh. I misread the episode as Shannon feeling inappropriately guilty, because she herself didn't racially abuse Romesh. But Shannon is a proud Nova Scotian, born and bred. Romesh is a racially visible minority group member, specifically recruited to increase diversity in our university faculty. Romesh suffered slights on more than one occasion because of the racial prejudice of Shannon's "people," and she felt guilty about it and felt the need to apologize. Shannon experienced what is known as "collective guilt"—the guilt that can come with the harmful actions of one's group or collective.

Everything we have looked at in this book so far has assumed that guilt is something that individual people have as a result of their own action, whether it is the feeling of guilt that comes from hurting a loved one, the guilt from sinning against God, or the legal guilt that comes from conviction for a crime. Romesh's experience and Shannon's reaction to it reveal that guilt can also come from the actions of a group, particularly when that group acts together. We might think of the abuse that Romesh suffered as the harmful actions of a few individuals, but it is also possible to see it as the product of a harmful collective attitude within a society that is racist or at least xenophobic. When I thought about the incident more, I was reminded of the crime from my youth. In court, when the trial judge had handed out similar sentences to the four of us even though we were charged with crimes of different seriousness, he had made a statement that ours was a group crime, and as such, we shared the guilt. Our crimes depended on the four of us acting together.* If the action and the harm that resulted depended on the existence of our group, then it makes sense to say that we were collectively guilty. In the same way, a society can be considered racist if it provides the conditions for individuals to express racism more easily.

But even if a group can *be* guilty of causing harm to others, why would a group member *feel* guilty if, like Shannon, they were not involved? We have seen throughout this book that the feeling of guilt is a self-conscious emotional experience. It arises from an assessment of our own role in causing harm to others. To the extent that we judge the self to be responsible for the harm, we will feel guilt. The

---

* Notwithstanding the judge's view on our crime, the law is generally not designed to manage collective guilt. It is an individual who is charged with a crime and an individual who is punished. That is why my sentence was reduced on appeal.

trick here is to consider how we conceive of our *self*. Take a moment to describe yourself. What descriptions do you use? Certainly, you will include your individual characteristics—probably both physical and psychological—but you will also likely include your group identities—perhaps your gender, your family, your ethnicity, your religion, your school or company, your nationality. For many people, the sense of self includes not just who they are as individuals, but also their social identity—who they are in terms of their social group memberships. Social identity in this sense can be a powerful organizing force in our individual psychology. You feel self-conscious emotions in reaction to your individual actions, but you may also feel them in reaction to the actions of the groups with which you identify. Think about how you feel when your country wins a gold medal in an Olympic event. You may not have had anything to do with that success, yet you may still feel proud. Just as we may feel pride in the achievements of our team, our school, our company, or our nation, so also we may feel guilt for their transgressions. And that is why Shannon felt guilty for how "her people" had treated Romesh.

One might ask why I did not feel the same collective guilt on hearing about Romesh's experience as Shannon. Part of the reason is that I do not identify as Nova Scotian to the same degree as she does. Although I have lived in this Canadian province for nearly forty years, I was not born here, did not grow up here, and my family are not from here. Being Nova Scotian is not a meaningful part of my self-concept and it probably never will be. When I meet Nova Scotians for the first time, they often hear my English accent and ask where I am from. If I am honest, I enjoy being "othered" in this way because I get to tell a small part of my personal story—where I grew up and why I emigrated to Canada. But perhaps of more significance is that I tend not to identify strongly with any groups. I prefer to think of myself as an individual rather than a group member, and as a consequence, while I feel a lot of personal guilt, I am generally free of collective guilt.*

Despite my own lack of feelings of collective guilt, there is no question that it plays an important role in our society, a role that arguably has grown over time to become very influential in contemporary

---

* And, by the same token, collective pride!

culture. Today, it is well accepted that groups, whether that is four undergraduate students or a nation of several million people, can share an objective collective guilt for their actions that cause harm to another group. It is also clear that individual members of those groups may feel guilt for the harm that their group has caused even if they had no personal involvement in causing that harm. These days, collective guilt drives personal behavior as well as institutional and public policy. Indeed, examining the role of collective guilt can help us understand many of the forces currently shaping our society. In this chapter, we will look in more detail at the origins of the idea of collective guilt and at some of the major areas in which it has become so salient. We start with the landmark event that keyed the world into the significance of collective guilt—the Holocaust.

German Guilt: The Guilt of a Nation and the Guilt of Its People

The time is December 1970, twenty-five years after the end of the Second World War. German Chancellor Willy Brandt is leading a delegation to Poland to sign a treaty recognizing a new western border of Poland, which will deprive some ethnic Germans of their territory. It is one act in Brandt's *Ostpolitik*, an olive branch foreign policy designed to rebuild East-West relations during the Cold War that will, within a year, earn him the Nobel Peace Prize. During the visit, Brandt makes a ceremonial stop at the memorial to the Warsaw Ghetto Uprising, commemorating the millions of Polish Jews who were murdered there and in the death camps by the Nazis. It's a typical gray early-winter day in northern Europe. There is a break in the cold rain as Brandt and the German delegation make their way toward the memorial. Brandt is solemn, his broad, square Slavic face revealing only that his thoughts are turned completely inwards. A large wreath is carried by two members of the delegation and placed against the top step of the memorial. Brandt slowly walks up to it and almost absent-mindedly adjusts the two wide ribbons in the colors of the German flag—black, red, and gold. He backs up, still looking at the wreath, and then falls, almost crumples, to his knees on the hard stone, his head tilted slightly forward. He remains in that position for about ten seconds as a hush falls on the assembled group of government officials, press corps, and survivors of the ghetto. Brandt then rises, turns slowly, and walks away from the memorial, still expressionless but now with his chin raised a little.

Brandt's gesture in front of the Warsaw Ghetto memorial, now known as the *Kniefall von Warschau,* or Warsaw genuflection, was a remarkable act in the history of international politics. It was an unprecedented sign of humility by a national leader, reflecting the posture of the sinner asking for forgiveness. By all accounts, the *Kniefall* was not planned. It was a spontaneous act from Brandt as the emotion of the event engulfed him. When later asked why he knelt in that way, he said, "All I could do was give a sign, to ask for forgiveness for my people, and pray that we might be forgiven."[1] As the political leader of Germany, Brandt was assuming the responsibility for his nation's guilt for its treatment of the Jews. And although we cannot know for sure, it seems from the way the *Kniefall* happened and his later explanation of it that Brandt himself felt this guilt personally.

Brandt's *Kniefall* was perhaps even more notable because he was in no way complicit with the crimes of Nazi Germany; indeed, he was an active opponent. Born Herbert Frahm to a working-class single mother in the German Empire city state of Lübeck in 1913, he joined the Social Democratic Party as a teenager and then the more left-wing Socialist Workers' Party (SAPD). As the Nazis rose to power in Germany during the 1930s, SAPD sympathizers were at risk of persecution, and he fled to Norway, adopting the pseudonym Willy Brandt to hide his identity from the Nazis. From there, he supported anti-Nazi causes and became a Norwegian citizen after the Nazis revoked his German citizenship. When the war ended, he returned to Germany and regained his German citizenship in 1946, now officially as Willy Brandt. He went on to build a significant career in politics, becoming mayor of West Berlin and then chancellor in 1969. Despite his opposition to the Nazis, as leader of the nation that had succumbed to Nazism and had caused such horrendous crimes, as a German, Brandt felt the guilt of those crimes.

The Holocaust and its aftermath was a watershed historical moment in the recognition that nations as a whole can be guilty for actions taken against groups of people based on their group identity.[2] The collective guilt lies in the harmful action being perpetrated by the group rather than by a particular individual or set of individuals. In Nazi Germany, there were countless degrees to which individuals were implicated in the persecution of the Jews. Some of these individuals were brought to justice. The Nazi leaders who were directly responsible for planning and orchestrating the war crimes were tried and convicted at the high-profile Nuremberg trials in 1945. A limited number of other lower-ranking members of the Nazis were sanctioned with fines and prison terms by a series of makeshift courts set up around the country by the Allies. But many people in Germany were complicit by acting under orders or even by turning a blind eye to what was going on around them, and most of them were never prosecuted. Put simply, the crimes of the Nazis could not have taken place without broad, organized, collective action. At Nuremberg and in local courts, certain individuals who enacted the Holocaust were brought to justice, but the nation as a whole was not.

But just as for individual guilt, collective guilt creates a need to resolve the guilt, to repair the relationships that have been harmed. It took the reorganization of German and Jewish interests into national-level issues to begin finally to resolve the relationship between Germany and the Jews. In 1948, the Zionist dream of nationhood was realized when Israel established its independence as a state.* Many of the Jews who remained in Germany as so-called displaced persons began to relocate to Israel. A year later, a new German nation—the Federal Republic of Germany (or West Germany) was established, and together, the two nations hammered out an agreement. West Germany admitted its guilt for the crimes against the Jews and agreed to pay reparations to the survivors of the Holocaust and to Israel, both to assist with the resettlement of Jewish refugees and to build the infrastructure and economy of that new nation. Certainly, this move by Germany has been seen as a form of *realpolitik,* or an expedient approach to rehabilitating its international credibility. Indeed, the German chancellor at the time, Konrad Adenauer, admitted as much. But the fact remains that Germany recognized its guilt and its responsibility for reparation and has

---

* It is, of course, tragically ironic that this resolution of the plight of the European Jews after the war initiated a new conflict in the Middle East—the Israel-Palestine conflict—for which collective guilt has again emerged.

continued to uphold that commitment to this day. Since the agreement was signed in 1952, over $70 billion has been paid by Germany to Israel.[3]

If progress had been made at the national level to repair the relationship between Germany and the Jews, what of the feelings of collective guilt that ordinary Germans experienced? It was the Swiss psychologist Carl Jung who coined the term "collective guilt" in a 1945 essay in which he suggested that it was inevitable that at some level, all Germans would feel guilt, even if they were not consciously aware of it.[4] Then, Theodor Adorno, a half-Jewish German philosopher who had spent much of the war in exile, carried out the first major study of the experience of collective guilt in 1950. He interviewed many ordinary German citizens of different ages and backgrounds about their collective responsibility for the Nazi crimes. The extent to which the study participants reported guilt varied according to how strongly they identified with their German identity. Adorno found that many of his respondents appeared to feel little guilt, arguing that there was little or nothing they could do about what had happened, and that Germans were no different from any other peoples. Other respondents were more open to expressing some guilt, accepting that they bore some responsibility for what had happened. These respondents were more supportive of providing compensation to the victims.[5]

Nevertheless, the progress in rebuilding West Germany into a democratic state proceeded through the two decades after the war with the defensiveness among its people toward the crimes of the Nazis relatively intact. Many Nazi officials were never prosecuted and even had their careers reborn in the West German bureaucracy.* Interestingly, it took a new generation of Germans, born after the war and therefore with no personal involvement in the crimes of the Nazis, to start to genuinely face up to the past. The initial significant upwelling of this collective guilt occurred with the first generation of Germans born after the war, who, as emerging adults in the 1960s, began to confront the reality that

---

* For example, it took almost twenty years for the justice system in Germany led by Fritz Bauer, a German lawyer who had spent part of the Nazi period in exile in Sweden and worked in the anti-Nazi resistance movement with Willy Brandt, to bring to trial the SS personnel who had murdered hundreds of thousands of Jews at Auschwitz.

their political leaders and even their parents shared some responsibility for the Holocaust. In 1968, West Germany, like other Western nations, was rocked by student protests. An important focus in Germany was that ex-Nazi sympathizers were still in powerful positions in the country. The chancellor at the time, Kurt Kiesinger, had himself been a member of the Nazi party, and was rumored to have been responsible for the deaths of ten thousand Greek Jews. The collective guilt in this new generation of Germans made a difference. The next year, Kiesinger lost the national election to Willy Brandt, who, as we have seen, was demonstrably not personally guilty of Nazi crimes. From that point on, the national conversation in Germany about the Nazi era became one of facing up honestly to the crimes of the past.

A decade later, a television event stimulated the next resurgence of collective guilt. *Holocaust*, an American television series depicting the events of the Holocaust through the eyes of a fictional Jewish family and an SS officer responsible for enacting the final solution, aired on German TV. Almost 40 percent of German households tuned into the series, an unprecedented viewing audience for such a show. *Holocaust* led to an intense round of public and private discussion about the Holocaust amongst a new generation of Germans. After the series had aired, polls showed that nearly 50 percent of the respondents reported shame for being German, and public sentiment in favor of compensation for the victims increased significantly.[6]

In his personal and insightful study of being Jewish in modern-day Germany, Yascha Mounk described how collective guilt for the crimes of the Nazis still impacts the lives of Germans and has led to two broad forms of reaction.[7] Many younger Germans engage in, and sometimes overindulge in, "philosemitism"—a professed admiration for the Jews. Mounk records the following interaction with a German friend:

> One morning, [Markus] greeted me with "*Chag sameach!*" in perfect Hebrew pronunciation.
>
> "Happy holidays to you, too," I replied. "But honestly, I don't even know what festival we have today."
>
> "The most important one. *Yom Kippur*. The Day of Atonement."
>
> "How do you know that?"
>
> "I learned about all the holidays for my bar mitzvah."

"Your bar mitzvah? I didn't realize you're Jewish."

"Well, I'm not really. Or rather, not anymore. I was for a few years, though. You see, when I was thirteen, I saw a documentary about the Holocaust. It devastated me. I felt so ashamed. I didn't know what I could do. So I converted to Judaism."

"But now you're not religious anymore?"

"I guess I just realized that it had all been a mistake."

"Because you never believed in God?"

"No, because I still feel guilty."

The other reaction is the desire among some Germans to "draw a line under the past." Unfortunately, some who insist on calling an end to collective guilt tend to do so in a passive-aggressive way, suggesting that it is the Jews who continue to bring up the past. For Mounk, at least, both reactions are unfortunate, because both overt philosemitism and overt or closet antisemitism continue to lead to an alienation of Germans and Jews from each other. In both cases, there is a failure to come together as equals. Mounk's account reveals that there is no natural way in which the collective guilt experienced by Germans can be dispelled through genuine forgiveness by those harmed. The groups remain apart, and many Jews like Mounk continue to feel like strangers in their own country.

Even today, guilt about the past remains an essential and important component of German national identity. But if the resolution of Germans' personal experience of collective guilt is challenging, the recognition of national collective guilt has motivated Germany to work to ensure that the kind of injustice perpetrated by their nation does not happen again. Certainly, like all countries, there is an undercurrent of nationalistic and xenophobic sentiment that sometimes bubbles to the surface,* but over the last fifty years, Germany has been a model for the integration of different groups into society. Indeed, according

---

* As I finalize these words in the summer of 2024, there is something of a wave of populist or nationalistic political resurgence occurring across Europe, including Germany.

to the United Nations, it has one of the most liberal and supportive immigration policies in the world.[8]

A New Era of Collective Guilt

The treatment of the Jews by Germany was horrendous, but it was far from the only episode in history where one group has systematically persecuted another. Group-on-group violence in the form of oppression, slavery, and genocide are common features of human history. Indeed, tribal violence and murder can be observed in our closest relatives in the animal world—chimpanzees—so it is surely not a recent development in human group relations.[9] Even as the events of the Second World War were unfolding, many other nations were simultaneously engaged in persecuting groups of their own citizens with devastating consequences for the victims. These nations included many of those fighting the Nazis. Nations created through colonization, including Canada, Australia, and New Zealand, were continuing their ongoing cultural genocide against Indigenous peoples. In the US, the legacy of slavery, which had been abolished in 1865, was still causing the discrimination and persecution of Black Americans under Jim Crow laws. Indeed, the American approach to treating ex-slaves and their descendants was viewed approvingly by the leadership of the Nazis, who adapted various aspects of Jim Crow legislation in their campaign to eliminate the Jews. The Nazis believed that their "solution" would have to be more drastic because, unlike American Black people at the time, who were struggling to rise in society and so could be more easily kept apart by discrimination alone, Jews in Germany were typically relatively wealthy, accomplished, and integrated into society.[10] Such harmful treatment of groups within their own countries continued relatively unexamined and unchecked even as these allies fought Nazism in Europe.

But something shifted in the way group persecution was viewed after the Holocaust. Perhaps it was the extreme and systematic nature of the Holocaust that focused the world's gaze on intergroup persecution; perhaps it was the historical coincidence with the development of mass media, including film and television, whereby images of the violence were available to everyone. The shock of the Holocaust led to a new perspective on intergroup relationships. The crime of "genocide" was instituted through an international treaty in the wake of the Second World War largely due to the advocacy of Raphael Lemkin, an American-based Polish Jewish lawyer who had lost family members in the Holocaust.[11] After the war, the spotlight, which had been shone on Nazi Germany, was inevitably turned toward other nations' treatment of their own citizens. Since then, the collective guilt of large groups such as nations, ethnic groups, religions, and cultures has grown to become a central focus of concern in the modern world. With the changes to international law, those groups that suffer oppression have legal and moral recourse to fight that oppression. Many groups responsible for oppression are now recognizing and accepting their collective guilt for their treatment of others and working on how to resolve it. Apologies, negotiations around reparations, and attempts at reconciliation have become commonplace, whereas prior to World War Two, they were almost unheard of.[12]

Settler Guilt

> I am sorry. I ask forgiveness, in particular, for the ways in which many members of the Church and of religious communities cooperated, not least through their indifference, in projects of cultural destruction and forced assimilation promoted by the governments of that time, which culminated in the system of residential schools.

With these words, during a visit to Maskwacis, Alberta in 2022, Pope Francis apologized to the Indigenous peoples of Canada for the Catholic Church's role in the country's residential school system. The apology was a recognition of guilt for the legacy of harm perpetrated on Indigenous peoples by the system of residential schools, in which the Catholic Church had played a central role.

As the Nazis were relocating Jewish citizens to ghettos and then preparing their final solution, the Government of Canada was engaged in a program of removal of Indigenous children from their families and relocating them to residential schools sometimes many kilometers away from their homes.* The residential school system in Canada became part of the national agenda with the Indian Act of 1876, not long after the birth of the country in 1867.[13] The main goal of the Indian Act was to assimilate Indigenous peoples into Euro-Canadian culture. For the new Canadian government, it was expedient and considerably less expensive to leave the operation of the schools to Christian religious orders that were experienced in providing missionary-based forms of education. The most active religious order in the administration of the residential schools was the Oblates of Mary Immaculate, a missionary branch of the Catholic Church, whose global vocation was to convert the natives of colonized lands to Christianity. Indeed, it was Vital-Justin Grandin, a Catholic bishop and leader of the Oblates of Mary Immaculate, who, in 1880, had helped convince the Government of Canada that the most effective means to assimilate the Indigenous population was to keep children away from their parents so they would forget "the customs, habits and language of their ancestors."[14]

At its height in 1931, the residential school system included eighty schools covering every region of Canada. The last was shuttered only in 1996. While the residential schools were in operation, some 150,000 Indigenous children were removed from their families. Forcible removal of children from their parents, families, and communities was bad enough, but the conditions the children experienced at the schools were deplorable—poor nutrition, strict rules denying the use of their native languages and culture, and regular physical and sexual abuse. Many children never made it home to their communities. Those that did carried with them the legacy of the abuses they suffered in high rates of health issues, such as diabetes, mental illness, including PTSD, substance abuse, and suicide. These harms have been passed on to subsequent generations through their damaging effects on family and community life, a phenomenon known as "intergenerational trauma." In Canada today, as in other countries, such as the US and Australia,

---

* The use of residential schools for cultural assimilation of Indigenous peoples was also introduced in the US in the nineteenth century and became widespread from the 1860s through the middle of the twentieth century. During the first half of the twentieth century, Australia also engaged in forced removal of Aboriginal children from their families, leading to what became known as the "Stolen Generations."

with Indigenous populations impacted by residential school systems, Indigenous people have significantly lower standards of living, suffer much higher rates of physical and mental health issues, and are much more likely to be incarcerated.

In the years after the Second World War, the idea of assimilation of one group by another became anathema in international law by its proximity to genocide. The Genocide Convention, which first codified genocide as a crime, defined it to include "forcibly transferring children of [one] group to another group." And although strictly speaking this was not the goal of the residential school system in Canada—in theory, the Indigenous children were to be returned to their communities after their "education"—forced assimilation certainly fits the notion of *cultural genocide*, an idea advanced by Raphael Lemkin, the Polish Jewish lawyer who first proposed the concept of the crime of genocide.

In the decades after the Genocide Convention, all the former European colonial nations began to review their relationships with their Indigenous peoples. Canada finally abandoned the forced assimilation policies of the Indian Act with the 1982 Constitution Act, which was designed to return the relationship between Canada and its Indigenous peoples to the idea inherent in the original treaties between King George III of England and the Indigenous peoples—a relationship of nation to nation—although this situation has still not yet been fully realized.[15]

While the Constitution Act of 1982 provided something of a reset for the relationship between Canada and its Indigenous peoples, it did not heal the harms that had been done while that relationship was disturbed. Abuse claims began to flood in from residential school survivors. These claims were handled through a consolidated response from Government[16] to a series of class action lawsuits from survivors. The government accepted its guilt and responded with by far the largest class action settlement in Canadian history, including approximately $1.9 billion in compensation to be distributed among all survivors, as well as a much larger allocation of over $3 billion for those with special claims of physical and sexual abuse. In 2008, the prime minister of the day, Stephen Harper, rose in the House of Commons to deliver a formal apology on behalf of the Government of Canada in recognition of the national guilt for the harm done to Indigenous peoples. This apology accompanied the initiation of a deep national soul-searching mission, the Truth and Reconciliation Commission (TRC), to turn the spotlight on the treatment of Canada's Indigenous peoples, to issue recommendations for how to heal the harms that had been perpetrated, and to work toward reconciliation between Indigenous peoples and the rest of Canada.[17]

The TRC report[18] was released in 2015 and, as one of its many recommendations, called upon the pope as the worldwide leader of the Catholic Church to make a formal apology for the role of the Catholic Church in the residential school system. The pope resisted this recommendation for some time, but repeated lobbying by the Government of Canada and Indigenous leaders finally led to the pope's formal apology, first in front of a delegation of Indigenous leaders who visited the Vatican City in April 2022, and then to multiple Indigenous communities during the pope's penitential pilgrimage to Canada in July 2022.

Whereas some were pleased to witness the pope's apology, others, including the chair of the Truth and Reconciliation Commission, Justice Murray Sinclair, expressed concern that it did not go far enough. As Justice Sinclair said in his response to the apology:

> Despite this historic apology, the Holy Father's statement has left a deep hole in the acknowledgment of the full role of the Church in the Residential School system, by placing blame on individual members of the Church. It is important to underscore that the Church was not just an agent of the state, nor simply a participant in government policy, but was a lead co-author of the darkest chapters in the history of this land.
>
> ...
>
> It was more than the work of a few bad actors—this was a concerted institutional effort to remove children from their families and cultures, all in the name of Christian supremacy.[19]

Why is it important that the pope acknowledge the role of the Catholic Church as an institution and not just of certain bad actors within it? For Justice Sinclair and other critics of the pope's apology, the responsibility and the guilt lie not just with the individuals who so mistreated the children in their care, but in the *institution* that promoted a religious and cultural colonial approach to that care. Justice Sinclair pointed out that there is a collective guilt of the Catholic Church that runs deeper than the guilt of the individual members of the Church who ran the residential schools. The harms to Indigenous children, including emotional, physical, and sexual abuse, were wrought by members of the Church within an overall approach to the treatment of Indigenous peoples that cast them as inferior, even less than human.

The colonial project legitimized both the assimilation of Indigenous peoples, which saw its nadir in Canada with the residential school system, and the claiming of colonized lands for over five hundred years. Only in the last few decades has the recognition of the collective guilt of colonization begun to be accepted. Those nations established through colonization have broadly begun to review their relationships with Indigenous peoples over the lands they inhabit. In Canada, as in other colonial nations, both of these aspects of colonization have begun to be addressed. Assimilation policies have been reversed. The TRC call for Indigenous culture to be taught in grade school as well as university courses, particularly in medicine and law, is being widely followed. Indigenous languages are being revived and taught more widely. The recognition and respect of land treaties remain hugely contentious. Although these land treaties were established between England and Indigenous nations during the reign of George III, they were subsequently ignored when Canada established itself as a nation. In recent years, Indigenous peoples in Canada, the US, Australia, and elsewhere have promoted the idea of "Land Back," a campaign to regain a degree of sovereignty and economic control over their traditional lands. But, of course, these lands have now been settled for generations by descendants of European colonizers as well as more recent immigrants like myself from many different nations, and there is no simple way to reach a resolution on land rights. There is at least a recognition of the problem in the widespread use of land acknowledgments. Land acknowledgments are not a solution, but by providing a constant reminder that the issue of treaty rights and self-governance are still not resolved in Canada, they are a start for reconciliation. The goal of course is to reach a place where efforts to resolve the national guilt will lead to full reconciliation and forgiveness.

Collective Guilt

White Guilt

> I don't remember hearing the phrase "white guilt" very much before the mid-sixties. Growing up black in the fifties, I never had the impression that whites were much disturbed by guilt when it came to blacks. When I would stray into the wrong restaurant in pursuit of a hamburger, it didn't occur to me that the waitress was unduly troubled by guilt when she asked me to leave. I can see now that possibly she was, but then all I saw was her irritability at having to carry out so unpleasant a task. If there was guilt it was mine for having made an imposition of myself.[20]

Since Black academic and author Shelby Steele was denied a hamburger in 1950s Chicago, the US has witnessed a remarkable change in race relations. In the 1950s, Jim Crow laws were still in effect. Segregation and discrimination based on race were explicitly woven throughout American legislation and culture, so much so that when Rosa Parks, a forty-two-year-old Black woman, refused to give up her seat on a Montgomery, Alabama, bus to a white man in 1955, she was arrested and charged with civil disobedience. As Steele suggests, guilt was likely not much of an issue for the white people who benefited from their society's cruelty toward Black Americans. Certainly, the nation was not ready to consider that it bore guilt for its history of racial oppression. But in the wake of the Holocaust, Rosa Parks's case and others like hers catalyzed a wave of civil rights activism from the Black community in America.

In this first phase of civil rights activism, the primary goal was to achieve individual human rights as well as economic benefits for Black Americans. Rosa Parks's refusal to give up her seat was a statement that she, as an individual, had just as much right to that seat as any white person. In his famous "I Have a Dream" speech delivered in 1963 at the March on Washington for Jobs and Freedom,[21] Martin Luther King Jr. referenced the American Declaration of ndependence and Constitution—the most individualistic statements of how to organize a nation ever conceived. As he said, "It is a dream deeply rooted in the American dream. I have a dream that one day this nation will rise up and live out the true meaning of its creed: 'We hold these truths to be self-evident, that all men are created equal.'" In perhaps the most moving line from his speech, King expressed his fervent wish that his "four little children will one day live in a nation where they will not be judged by the color of their skin but by the content of their character." It was King, a Baptist minister, who, more than anyone else, convinced mainstream America that civil rights was a moral issue and that, despite the Founding Fathers' eloquent words, their nation had been collectively guilty of denying those rights to Black people throughout its history. His solution was to move beyond treating people according to their collective racial group and to treat everyone as an equal individual. The result was the passage of the Civil Rights Act of 1964, which made discrimination and segregation based on race illegal.

Beginning with the Civil Rights Act, the US began to work on its national collective guilt.* Under the banner of "The Great Society," President Lyndon B. Johnson introduced a series of federal policies that included changes to voting rights, as well as investments in education, housing, welfare, and health care. In principle, The Great Society policies were supposed to be nondiscriminatory—the benefits were not based on race but on need. But these benefits were to be used as the main tool to dismantle discrimination and segregation because they could be withheld if jurisdictions maintained discriminatory policies. And, because of the widespread inequality favoring white people over Black people, those federal benefits were intended to flow to a greater extent to Black people in need. The investments of The Great Society policies did not have the intended effect of significantly reducing racial economic disparities, in part because of the economic demands made by the Vietnam War. So-called affirmative action policies were introduced in the 1960s to ensure fair and equal access to education and jobs. While designed to redress historical discrimination, affirmative action has been more controversial. Because the assessment of equal access involved monitoring equal outcomes, some argued that affirmative action became in effect reverse discrimination, with differential

---

* There had been earlier legal cases that had begun to address racial discrimination, most notably the 1954 Supreme Court decision in *Brown v. Board of Education of Topeka* that declared school segregation unconstitutional, but the Civil Rights Act was the landmark legislation that was designed to dismantle all racial discrimination.

standards applying to different racial groups. Challenges to this practice have ensued, and as a result, affirmative action is now illegal in certain jurisdictions. In 2023, the US Supreme Court ruled that the use of affirmative action in university admissions was unconstitutional.

Alongside policies designed to address racial inequality, various levels of government have issued apologies for the historic treatment of Black people. In 2008, the US Congress passed a resolution apologizing for slavery and the history of discriminatory laws. Various states have issued similar apologies, and even some large cities, including Boston and San Francisco, have followed suit. While well-meaning, it is difficult to see how these apologies can be useful. The problem, of course, is that there is no obvious path for forgiveness to take place. Governments may speak for the perpetrator of systemic racism, but when it comes to racial discrimination, there is no forum or representative of those harmed to accept the apology. As a result, these apologies have little power to effect reconciliation.

The Civil Rights Act and the suite of Great Society policies that followed did not magically wash away racist attitudes or racial inequalities. In fact, attitudes toward racial integration actually deteriorated between 1963 and 1966, as evidenced by polls conducted at the time.[22] Overt racism and substantial support for racial segregation persisted throughout the 1960s and into the 1970s, particularly in the southern states, but also in working-class white neighborhoods in the North that resisted integration. For example, George C. Wallace, the Democratic governor of Alabama, vocally opposed desegregation in the lead-up to the passage of the Civil Rights Act, and ran for president as an independent with a segregation platform in 1968, securing electoral college votes from six Southern states, a feat not achieved since for an independent candidate.* Through this period, Black activists began more and more to reject the individualism and passivism of Martin Luther King Jr. in favor of promoting the interests of Black people as a group. Under the banner of Black Power, Black nationalist groups such as the Nation of Islam and the Black Panthers took up the fight for Black rights. This wave of activism was influential in normalizing the idea that

---

* By the late 1970s, Wallace had become a born-again Christian, renounced segregationist views, and apologized to Black Americans.

American society had always been and continues to be racist. Sixty years on from the passage of the Civil Rights Act, racial inequalities in the US are still broad and deep. Inequalities favoring white people over Black people can be seen today in educational achievement, financial resources and standard of living, incarceration rates, and so on. In the present day, systemic racism can be seen in the frequency of police violence against Black people and in superficially color-blind policies such as the War on Drugs that have had a profoundly discriminatory effect and wreaked enormous differential damage to Black communities. The War on Drugs is the foremost reason why Black Americans today are incarcerated at much higher rates than whites.[23] The activism based on collective racial identity also normalized the idea that racial disparities are best addressed by reference to group identity rather than individual rights. In contemporary America, this identity politics approach is represented by influential voices such as Ta-Nehisi Coates[24] and Ibram X. Kendi[25] as well as activist organizations such as Black Lives Matter (BLM). In their view, the guilt of historic and contemporary systemic racism has created an enduring debt to Black people that still needs to be paid. For example, Ta-Nehisi Coates has written eloquently about the economic discrimination endured by Black people since the end of slavery and the case for reparations.[26] As Ibram X. Kendi put it in his bestselling book *How to Be an Antiracist*, "[T]he only remedy to past discrimination is present discrimination. The only remedy to present discrimination is future discrimination." In this view, where there are inequalities based on race, resources, including educational and employment opportunities, health care, and public housing, should be preferentially allocated based on race. To take one example, when it emerged that Black people had higher hospitalization and mortality rates than white people during the Covid-19 pandemic, a strong argument was made by many in the health care system that race should be a factor in allocating scarce vaccines and antiviral medications.[27]

But not everyone agrees with the identity politics approach to solving racial inequities. The modern heirs to Martin Luther King Jr.'s individualism, including Black authors such as Shelby Steele,[28] John McWhorter,[29] and Coleman Hughes,[30] are typically more sanguine about the progress that has been achieved in the last sixty years toward a racially fair society.* These authors recognize the reality of inequality but believe that significant progress has been made, that the US is no longer systemically racist, and that the march toward true equality is on track, even if behind schedule. They argue that an individualist or "color-blind" approach still offers the best hope of a genuinely racially fair society. McWhorter, for example, has argued that major strides toward reducing racial inequality would be achieved by policies such as abandoning the War on Drugs, and the provision of high-quality early education for all children. Furthermore, these voices argue that the calls for antiracist discrimination that advocates like Kendi and Coates promote are counterproductive for achieving true equality. As an example, Steele focuses on how affirmative action has created a situation where Black success comes with an asterisk—success is achieved through a helping hand rather than through merit—and in the long run, this will harm Black people.

Clearly, these are not easy issues to resolve, and certainly, as a psychologist, I am not qualified to suggest how best to fix the racial inequalities and finally discharge the debt created by the crimes of slavery and subsequent societal discrimination.[31] Whether the solution to racial inequalities will come through interventions preferentially targeting Black people, through interventions designed to reduce all inequalities, or through the arrangement of a society free of all discrimination and intervention are primarily political, sociological, and economic questions. But I can suggest how the collective guilt experienced by white people works in this environment of racial inequality.

At the outset, I need to be clear on what we mean by "white guilt" and who experiences it. White guilt is the experience of guilt that people may have in connection with their membership in the racial group—white people—responsible for historical and contemporary oppression of Black people. Patrick Grzanka and his colleagues at the University of Tennessee adapted the TOSCA measure of guilt-proneness that we looked at in Chapter 2 to assess white guilt specifically.[32] When they gave their new measure to a large sample of white

---

* These authors are often referred to as "conservative," but it may be more accurate to describe them as classically liberal, in the sense of adhering to a political philosophy that prioritizes the individual over the collective.

Americans, they found that white guilt does not affect everyone equally. Certain demographics of the US population were much more likely to report guilt in connection with race relations. We should not be surprised to learn that women report more white guilt overall than men, given that they report more guilt in general. But, in addition, the researchers found that participants who self-identified as Democrats expressed more white guilt than those who self-identified as Republicans or independents. So, guilt over race relations appears to be more associated with a left-leaning political identity than with being white *per se*.*

As an advocate for the idea that guilt can be a good thing, it is interesting to me that none of those debating how to counteract racial inequality seems to have much good to say about white guilt.[33] For example, Ibram X. Kendi has no time for the feelings of guilt that whites experience. He suggests this white guilt leads to largely unhelpful performative activism. A significant engine for this guilt is the fear of being thought or called racist, and of being shunned by one's peer group because of it. Here, guilt originates in the fear of the loss of one's relationships with others in the peer group—typically a left-leaning community concerned with social justice. Those who are driven by this fear are mostly concerned with defending against the appearance of racism. They may react with what might be considered largely worthless performative activism, such as holding BLM signs at demonstrations after the murder of George Floyd or listing #BLM in their social media profiles. They may also show anger (sometimes termed "moral outrage") toward those they perceive to be insufficiently motivated to end racism. But they do little else to work toward racial equality. This form of white guilt does little substantively to improve the lives of Black people. As Ibram X. Kendi says about attending demonstrations:

> We convince ourselves we are doing something to satisfy our feelings. We go home fulfilled, like we dined at our favorite restaurant....The problems of inequity and injustice persist. They persistently make us feel bad and guilty. We persistently do something to make ourselves

---

* So, one might cheekily term this form of guilt "white progressives' guilt"!

feel better as we convince ourselves we are making society better, as we never make society better. *What if instead of a feelings advocacy we had an outcome advocacy that put equitable outcomes before our guilt and anguish?* What if we focused our human and fiscal resources on changing power and policies to actually make society better, not just our feelings better?[34]

If Kendi suggests white guilt is pointless, Shelby Steele is even more damning. He suggests that the feeling of white guilt that has permeated liberal America since the widespread recognition of the sin of racial discrimination has created an unfortunate, paternalistic approach to dealing with racial inequality that has actively harmed Black people by positioning them constantly as victims. He writes, "White guilt was a smothering and distracting kindness that enmeshed minorities more in the struggle for white redemption than in their own struggle to develop as individuals capable of competing with all others."[35] Steele's words here echo a line from the speech delivered in 1966 by Martin Luther King Jr. at Soldier Field, Chicago: "The white man needs the Negro to free him from his guilt."[36] For Steele, white guilt is actively harmful to the struggle for racial equality.

While I can see the concerns that authors such as Kendi and Steele express, as a psychologist (and white person), I would like to offer a perspective on white guilt that suggests it has some value. I am not as dismissive of the value of white guilt as these authors are. In general, psychological research on collective guilt has shown that those who report feeling collective guilt are more favorably inclined toward the victims of group-on-group harm, are in favor of apologies by the leaders to the victims of group harm, and are more supportive of policies aimed at reducing inequality, such as affirmative action and reparations, than those who do not experience collective guilt.[37] Studies of young adults have shown that those who report more white guilt are more likely to engage in various forms of civic action, such as voting, volunteering, and community engagement.[38] So, collective guilt provides an important foundation for a generally positive attitude toward improving race relations. President Joe Biden recognized this when, in a speech to convince Congress to pass the Freedom to Vote bill, designed to remove barriers to voting for Black Americans, in January 2022, he asked members of Congress whether they wanted to be on the side of Martin Luther King Jr. or George Wallace, a quite naked attempt to induce guilt in those considering opposing the bill.[39]

However, the devil is in the details because, as we know, guilt is not a simple emotion. The feeling of guilt involves fear of relationship loss, empathy for those harmed, and remorse for one's role in causing harm. Guilt also comes directly from hurting someone we care about and from contravening our conscience. Each of these elements can play into the reaction to racial inequality differently. I have already suggested that one source of white guilt, particularly for a left-leaning demographic, is the fear of relationship loss among one's peer group, and this is of minimal value in promoting racial equality. As Kendi says, it prioritizes attempts to minimize the perception of racism rather than constructive attempts to dismantle it. Guilt may also be stimulated by empathy for those harmed, but empathy is a reaction that tends to occur when encountering the harms suffered by individuals, not the systemic harms experienced by the group as a whole. A clear example of guilt based primarily on empathy was seen in the reaction to the horrific video footage of George Floyd's murder in June 2020. This event caused not only mass outrage from Black Americans, but also an outpouring of white guilt. Like the guilt based on the fear of being thought racist, guilt based predominantly on empathy for Floyd led to considerable performative activism manifested as expressions of grief for the victim and anger against the police perpetrators (extended to the police in general for crimes against Black victims). Again, this activism may serve primarily to reduce the guilt rather than drive the change needed at a systemic level.

I believe that when it comes to counteracting racial inequality, there is more value in guilt that is primarily based on remorse for one's role in maintaining inequality. Remorse is the self-focused aspect of guilt. It occurs when one accepts that one has a degree of responsibility for the harm that has occurred. Even if whites believe they have not directly acted in a racist way, nevertheless they may accept that they enjoy the benefits of unearned privilege at the expense of Black people. And this recognition of inequity contravenes standards of conscience, which generates guilt. Psychological research has shown that for white Americans, a strong belief in the reality of unearned white privilege is associated with greater feelings of guilt.[40] Furthermore, in studies where white Americans are led to focus either on their own white privilege or on the disadvantages that minorities experience, guilt is stronger in those that focus on white privilege.[41]

It is fair to say that sixty years on from the passage of the Civil Rights Act, the US remains a nation that, even if it has recognized its collective guilt for the history of crimes against Black people, has failed to resolve that guilt. Racial inequities remain stark, and the solution to these inequities seems as elusive as ever. Nevertheless, the collective guilt of white people likely has to be a part of that solution. Only by taking responsibility for the continuing harms suffered by Black people can progress toward dismantling the destructive legacy of racial discrimination be maintained.

Green Guilt

Let's return to the other appearance of guilt in the story with which I opened this chapter. As I sat in the idling car, waiting for Shannon to finish checking up on Romesh and his washing machine, I felt a familiar twinge of guilt. I knew I really shouldn't be letting the car idle, even if it was getting chilly. It gnawed at my conscience, but, I'm sorry to say, not enough to make me turn it off. For me, as for many people, these micro-episodes of "eco-guilt" or "green guilt"—the guilt associated with acting in a way that is not environmentally responsible—occur constantly. I get them when I don't bring my own cup to the coffee shop at work, when I leave the water running as I brush my teeth, when I forget to turn off the light in a room I have exited. It seems these days that everyday life is a minefield of guilt because so much of what we do can be examined in terms of its impact on the health of the planet. The food we eat, the clothes we wear, the way we get around, the vacations we enjoy, all present a challenge to living a sustainable life. It is all too common to feel guilt that we are not doing enough to save the planet.

My experience is corroborated by the explosion of books, articles, and blogs on green guilt in the last twenty years.[42] According to one US national survey in 2015, more than a third of respondents reported feeling green guilt.[43] If adults in general are becoming preoccupied with green guilt, the concern is even greater in today's younger generation. A recent survey asked ten thousand adolescents and young adults from ten countries from around the globe[44] about their feelings regarding the climate crisis. Over two-thirds said they were afraid of what the future holds for them, and more than 50 percent said they felt guilty. Given that, in their short lives, they had made minimal contributions to global warming, these young people appear to be experiencing a form of collective guilt for the way their species has treated the planet. In a direct test of this idea, Mark Ferguson and Nyla Branscombe measured green guilt in American university students who were told either that global warming was caused by human activity or was the result of natural processes.[45] They found that the students who had been told about human causes of global warming reported more guilt than those who had been told about natural causes of global warming. This guilt also made them express more positive opinions about conserving energy and paying an additional tax on gasoline.

But why do we feel *guilt* about harming the planet if guilt is primarily about managing social relationships? In part, it is a matter of conscience. That is what I experienced in the car that night. Like many of my generation, I was steeped by my parents in a culture of not being wasteful and of reusing everything. In part, this was their reaction to the austerity born in the war years. But it quickly morphed into a concern for the environment during the 1960s, when books such as Rachel Carson's *Silent Spring*, which highlighted the damage pollution was doing to the environment, captured the public imagination.[46] Responsibility for the environment, sometimes captured in the "3 Rs" (reduce, reuse, recycle) became embedded in cultural and even ethical norms for my generation and those that followed. We came to understand as a community that taking action to reduce consumption, limit waste, and use less energy is the right thing to do.

But there is an additional source of green guilt these days. As concerns about pollution have transitioned into concerns about climate change and global warming, the urgency of environmental responsibility has become even greater. And this responsibility is not just to the environment, but to the groups of people that will be harmed by our current irresponsibility. In fact, global warming is potentially the most extreme case of group-on-group harm the world has ever seen. Climate change has now succeeded pollution or concerns about nuclear war as the most significant environmental and existential threat to humanity. Climate change is on track to cause the mass destruction of the habitat and lifestyles of future generations by those alive today. The gradual rise in global temperature since the Industrial Revolution and the future trajectory of that increase suggests that while I will see some limited impacts during the remainder of my life, major impacts will be experienced by my child, who was born in 1999, and by my potential grandchildren. Where I live in Nova Scotia, global warming will likely lead to significant sea level rise as the glaciers of the world melt and the land mass sinks. At the same time, ever more violent hurricanes spawned in the Caribbean will work their way up the North American Eastern Seaboard, causing damage to natural habitats and human settlements. Sea level rise and intensifying storm surges could well result in Nova Scotia becoming an island in less than one hundred years.[47]

On a global scale, the damage will be enormous. Worldwide, hundreds of millions of people live in coastal areas that are at severe risk of flooding and irreversible destruction from sea level rise.[48] Take the island nation of the Maldives, sitting just two meters above sea level in the Indian Ocean. Approximately half a million Maldivians could be forced to flee their country by the end of this century if sea level rise meets the predictions of the Intergovernmental Panel on Climate Change (IPCC). Many more people worldwide will be affected by shifts in weather patterns that will ramp up the heat waves, droughts, and wildfires that have become more common in the last decade. In short, many people around the globe will see their homes and livelihoods impacted and, in many cases, ruined. Now, because global warming is a planetary phenomenon, those who will suffer the severest consequences are not necessarily those most responsible for the harm caused by carbon emissions. Historically, it has been the industrialized First World nations that have produced the bulk of the carbon released into the atmosphere. Currently, the US and China are the largest emitters. Yet many poorer countries will take the brunt of the damage. As I write this chapter, the issue of climate compensation for countries most affected by global warming is on the agenda of COP27 in Egypt. While the debate has been careful to avoid assigning guilt or blame, referring only to compensation for "loss and damage," it is clear that the responsibility for global warming and the harm it will wreak on poorer nations is now being accepted by those nations that have been the major contributors to climate change.

For many people of an older generation who will witness relatively little impact from global warming in their lifetimes (like me), the feeling of guilt arises more from a consideration of how their actions will damage their relationship with those who will be most affected by the climate emergency: future generations. It is telling that the person who established perhaps the most influential platform to spread the message of the climate emergency in the last ten years began her activism as a child. At the age of fifteen, Greta Thunberg organized the first school strike in Sweden to protest climate inaction. She has gone on to become one of the most recognized activists in the world, was named *Time* magazine's "Person of the Year" in 2019,[49] and has been nominated for the Nobel Peace Prize. Her message was grounded in anger at how those who are in control today are harming those who will follow by not doing enough to prevent the irreversible planetary damage that can be foreseen only too well. Thunberg's appeal was not so much in drawing the world's attention to the effects of climate change. Many before her, including many of the world's climate scientists, had done that to limited fanfare. She drew the world's attention to *who* would be most affected—her generation and those that followed. Framing the climate emergency in terms of the harm it will cause to our children and their children is the most powerful way to elicit guilt in those in a position to create change today. In a sense, parental guilt wears the cloak of green guilt.

So, what can be done about this guilt? As with the other forms of collective guilt we have reviewed in this chapter, the resolution of green guilt is difficult. We know that true resolution requires forgiveness, and there is no obvious route to forgiveness when those who are most harmed are the future inhabitants of the planet. But even if forgiveness by those who will be harmed is impossible, the responsibility for mitigating the harm remains, and this responsibility requires both individual and collective action. While their contribution to global greenhouse gas emissions is significantly lower than that of industry and agriculture, individual households, particularly through vehicle use and home heating and cooling, are not negligible sources of the greenhouse gases that contribute to global warming. As a result, there has been a lot of research directed at ways to motivate people to reduce their energy footprint.[50] Guilt has emerged as a particularly important psychological factor in moving people to engage in more environmentally friendly behavior. For example, Ian Adams and his colleagues gave a sample of US Americans an assessment of their carbon footprint by asking them about their energy use.[51] They then gave them feedback telling them they were either high or low carbon emitters compared to the general population. Then they measured how guilty they felt. At a one-week follow-up, participants were asked to estimate how much they had engaged in various environmentally friendly behaviors, such as turning off lights when leaving a room. The results showed that those who were told their carbon footprint was high showed more green behaviors during the follow-up period and that this was directly related to how much guilt they reported. Even if I didn't switch off the engine that cold night while waiting for Shannon, there are plenty of times when my green guilt does lead me to limit my energy use.

So, it seems that making people aware of their contributions to carbon emissions can stimulate guilt and can lead them to be more responsible. Companies selling carbon offsets have recognized this dynamic for a while. A few years ago, the travel company Travelocity would respond to customers purchasing an airline ticket with the following offer to buy carbon credits: "Effectively offset the negative environmental impact of your entire trip. Go without guilt—Go Zero!"[52] And Carbonfund.org now offers the opportunity to purchase carbon offsets to neutralize the carbon impact of one's whole life for the price of US$20,400.[53]

Green guilt has become widespread in the twenty-first century. And, even if it is uncomfortable, let's hope it stays that way. It offers the best chance we have for mitigating, if not completely averting, the climate crisis heading our way, and securing a healthy planet for our children and their children.

Collective guilt is both an objective reality, akin to criminal guilt, of groups that have perpetrated harm on other groups, and a subjective experience of members of those groups that have perpetrated the harm. Beginning with the aftermath of the Holocaust, the last eighty years have witnessed an unprecedented willingness for large-scale collectives such as nations or religions to recognize and accept their guilt in perpetrating harms on other groups. The guilt arises because, as with individual guilt, relationships have been harmed. With collective guilt, it is the relationships between groups—between Germans and

Jews, between European Canadians and Indigenous peoples, between white and Black Americans, and between the current generation of humans and their children and their children's children—that have been harmed. The guilt of group members plays an important role in motivating those groups to do better. As when an individual harms another person with whom they have a relationship, apology and reparations can serve to heal the harms and restore relationships between the groups. It took many years, but Germany has come a long way in its journey to restore its relationship with the Jewish people. Other nations that have recognized their collective guilt are still in the early stages of reconciliation. Nevertheless, the acceptance of this guilt is a critical step. It is the foundation for instituting the process of reconciliation even if determining the particular means by which to achieve reconciliation after many years of harm may be challenging.

As Willy Brandt so famously illustrated, members of groups that have harmed other groups experience guilt from the actions of their collectives even if as individuals they did nothing wrong. This guilt arises because affinity with our social groups is a fundamental aspect of our identity formation. The guilt of members of a group that has caused harm to another group remains a key piece of the path to reconciliation. In the end, it is what will motivate people to create change in their society to compensate for the harms that their group has caused and, hopefully, to prevent such harms from occurring again.

Part III Takeaways

Human societies involve networks of relationships that extend far beyond those close to us or those with whom we regularly interact. Nevertheless, guilt is there to manage these relationships just as it does for our everyday relationships. When harm occurs in relationships that are not personal, the subjective experience of guilt may be less relevant. We just don't naturally care in the same way for people we do not know well. But the reduced experience of guilt that comes when we harm those distant from us may be supplemented by other forms of guilt. When it comes to harm to relationships that lack a personal nature, there is a much more significant role for the guilt that conscience delivers and for the objective guilt of societal rules.

Religious guilt can be thought of as the transformation of the guilt endemic to communal relationships into a wider societal guilt. In particular, the Abrahamic religions introduced a broader notion of family with all members of the religion united under one God. God is the father figure whose rules for how to behave and for how to treat others provide the guidance on how to live one's life—in effect, the societal version of the conscience that we all acquire through our early interactions with our parents. Because the believer has a relationship with God—whether direct for Christians or more mediated by the prophet Muhammad for Muslims—guilt may be experienced directly when God's laws are transgressed. And it is this guilt that keeps the believer in line with their faith. When the believer steps out of line, there is a clear path to forgiveness and restoration of the relationship with God through the expression of contrition. So, the resolution of guilt is integrated fully into the practice of religion.

Legal systems take the religious approach to the provision of rules for appropriate behavior in society even further. In the law, rules are codified in detail and, in the absence of a parental figure who is to be obeyed to protect the relationship, the legal system provides a focus, essentially entirely, on whether those rules have been contravened and what the repercussions are. But the focus on the protection of the integrity of society rather than the relationship between those committing crime and their victims can often mean that when guilt is determined, it is difficult to achieve forgiveness and genuine reconciliation.

Religions and legal systems are there to provide guidance for individuals on how to live their lives and manage their relationships. With collective guilt, we move to the ways in which individuals and the larger social groups of which those individuals are members interact. Groups of people have relationships too, and these relationships often get disrupted. For most of history, it was reasonable to say that guilt was not a factor in group relationships. Perhaps we could liken such group relationships to exchange relationships between individuals—to the extent there was interaction, it was more about getting the best deal out of the other, even if that meant exploitation, pain, and suffering for the other. But in the middle of the twentieth century, a much more communal idea of intergroup relationships took root. It is now widely considered unacceptable for one group to exploit or persecute another. Guilt has very much become a factor, both in the sense that a group as a whole can bear guilt for its actions toward another group and in the sense that members of a group can feel guilty for the actions of their group. This introduction of guilt into the management of intergroup relations is of profound importance to the health of the global community.

Conclusion

Making Friends with Guilt

A long time ago, I had a crash course on guilt and its resolution. It launched me on a lifelong journey to understand guilt and its role in human experience. I have tried to lay out what I have learned in this book. In this final chapter, I want to leave with a simple message: we need to be *making friends with guilt*. I mean this phrase in two senses.

First, I mean that we need to recognize and to value the real purpose of guilt. I have argued throughout this book that guilt is mostly beneficial, that it is the best guide we have for managing our relationships when they are challenged. But guilt has an image problem. Nobody wants to *feel* guilt.[1]

No one wants to feel guilt because it is so unpleasant. It is part fear and anxiety, part sadness, and part anger. On their own, each of these emotions is unpleasant; together, they're awful. But there's a good reason we feel negative emotions: they move us to act to protect ourselves and to protect others. Think about pain. No one likes to be in pain, but pain is important and helpful—it signals to us when there might be tissue damage. If we didn't feel pain, we would suffer many more bruises, cuts, burns, and all forms of bodily damage. Pain motivates us to protect our bodies from injury and repair harm that has occurred. In the case of guilt, its purpose is to signal that we may have put our relationships at risk, and we should do something to protect and heal them. We saw in Chapter 4 what happens when guilt is absent. Lacking the emotions that form guilt, psychopaths treat others purely as a means to satisfy their own ends. They develop few if any deep, meaningful relationships, and their lives often descend into a pattern of harming others and, in the long run, themselves. So, the capacity for guilt says something good about you. It means that you care about others. It means that you value your relationships with them.

And it means you regret it when you hurt them. These are all positive statements about who you are as a person and as a member of society. So, the next time you feel guilt, embrace what it is telling you.

I think a big reason for guilt's image problem is its association with the idea of *being* guilty. No one wants to be guilty, because being guilty means you have broken the rules that govern our lives, a fact that often entails disapproval and punishment. These rules begin during our early upbringing. Misbehaving as children leads to parental censure and sometimes the threat of punishment. As adults, we think of guilt in terms of criminality: to be guilty under the law is to have broken the law and committed a crime. The criminal justice system approach to guilt is typically retributive. If we're guilty of a crime, then the repercussion is usually punishment and the stigma of being a convicted felon. Making good on how we may have harmed others is often more of an afterthought. For those who are religious, guilt means sin, over which hangs the threat of punishment for being unworthy of God's love. Too often, we transfer this punitive approach to the feeling of guilt in our everyday personal lives. We think that if we feel guilt, then we deserve to be punished. This is a mistake; feeling guilt should be a spur to make things right, not a scourge to stigmatize us in our own and others' eyes.

Although guilt should be about *what one did*, too easily, the feeling of guilt can devolve into a judgment of *who one is*. This conflation of action with actor plagues us all in society. We think of guilt as a property of criminals, of sinners, of bad sorts. A judgment of character of this kind suggests the likelihood of further wrongdoing. We assume the guilty are more likely than the innocent to be guilty again in the future. So, guilt can be reputational poison. What we forget is that, sometimes, assuming that guilt should be attributed to people rather than to actions can become a self-fulfilling prophecy. Bad people will, of course, do bad things again; good people who do bad things can learn to do better.

So, let's accept guilt as a necessary and important part of the human condition. Let's think of guilt as a positive and healthy emotion, because even though it feels bad, it serves to mend damaged relationships. If we take this approach to guilt, then the default reaction to feeling guilt will be: What can I do to make my relationships better? And this takes us to the second sense of making friends with guilt: we should use guilt to enhance our relationships.

Conclusion

We all need a network of relationships to lead happy and fulfilled lives. At the core of this network are those communal relationships that are most meaningful to us—in most cases, our natal family, the family we may acquire through romantic relationships, and a circle of close friends. Beyond that core, relationships characterize the human condition, from individuals to nations. Some of these relationships are given to us, some we choose, but all can be at risk of damage when we act, as we almost inevitably will at some point, in ways that are selfish and uncaring.

Guilt is the best signal we have that we need to work on our relationships. When we feel it, we should pay attention and use it as a guide. Sometimes, this means owning up to a transgression and apologizing. There's no better way to restore a relationship than to make an authentic apology—*sorry* really shouldn't be the hardest word! Even if we didn't do anything wrong or hurtful, guilt can mean that we just haven't put in the effort to nurture the relationship. Sometimes, dealing with guilt just means showing the other some TLC.

I should note that I am not suggesting that guilt is infallible as a signal that our relationships need some work. For those who are particularly guilt-prone or who are caring for someone who is dependent, such as a child or aging parent, guilt can sometimes get out of hand and become counterproductive. This situation is especially common when the one being cared for is not able to let you know that you are, in fact, caring enough. It's important to remember that guilt is an emotion, not a rational thought process. Guilt is triggered by circumstances that suggest relationship threat, such as a loved one being upset, and it needs to be supplemented by a rational assessment of one's responsibility. So, when we feel guilt, it is always worth assessing honestly to what extent we are responsible for the harm, or potential harm, that someone else may be experiencing.

This kind of assessment of responsibility is also important when we find ourselves in the more toxic circumstances where someone we care about is guilt-tripping us. Guilt induction is an effective tool for manipulation of caring people. Sometimes, it is a reasonable strategy within a relationship to help modify or train a friend's or a partner's behavior, but it can also be used to excess. Those who tend to be relatively anxious in relationships worry about the health of their relationships constantly. This anxiety primes the tendency to feel guilt and makes them vulnerable to the guilt trip. If you find you are constantly feeling guilty in your relationships despite your best efforts to be caring, then it may not be you but your partner who is at fault.

This mention of the guilt trip should remind us that communal relationships are ideally a two-way street. Both partners should give and receive care. And when the health of the relationship is challenged, both partners should participate in its restoration, no matter who was at fault. Ideally, guilt will move one person to try to mend a damaged relationship, but healing can only come with forgiveness by the harmed party. So, as the great religions of the world teach us, there is an onus on the one who has been harmed to forgive. That's not to say forgiveness should be unconditional. The harmed party is owed some reassurance that the harm will not reoccur. But still, if a relationship is worth keeping, then both parties need to bend toward the other for it to work.

What, then, of situations where forgiveness is not forthcoming, as when a partner refuses to forgive or perhaps is no longer available to forgive? If guilt's purpose is to effect reconciliation, then it is important to know when to let go of it. This is often easier said than done because regret can be pernicious and long-lasting. In such circumstances, self-forgiveness is important. How do we self-forgive? One useful trick is to imagine if the roles in the relationship were flipped. If you are unable to achieve forgiveness from the other, imagine what you would do if the roles were reversed. Would you forgive someone you cared about if they had done what you did but then felt genuine remorse and apologized? If you could see your way to forgiving them, then it only makes sense for you to forgive yourself.

If guilt is such a good thing, then why does it sometimes become unhealthy? For reasons we have explored, guilt can become excessive and too difficult to manage on one's own. Excessive guilt can come from overly harsh parenting, particularly at an early age, or from events that result in the traumatic severance of a relationship. Under these conditions, we may not even recognize the underlying guilt for what it is. It is masked by anxiety and self-loathing, and so it can be difficult to manage on one's own. Then, therapeutic assistance may be critical for exposing the guilt and how it is rooted in disrupted relationships. Again, identifying the guilt and its origin in damaged relationships can become the key to unlock and alleviate the mental distress. Even in cases when guilt becomes debilitating, targeting the resolution of the guilt feelings can offer a way back to psychological health.

If there is one lesson that I would want this book to convey, it is that guilt needs to shed its image problem. Yes, guilt is horrible, but like the best medicines of old, it is good for you. It helps us to identify when our relationships may be at risk, and it guides us to work on them and to restore them. Caring for our relationships, from the intimate to the global, is the most important task we face in life. So, let's welcome guilt into our lives and make friends with it. Our relationships, and indeed our society, will be stronger for it.

Acknowledgments

In a sense I have been working on this project for all my adult life but the roots of the book really took hold when I was enrolled in the MFA program at the University of King's College in Halifax, Nova Scotia, from 2020–2022. I thank Kim Pittaway for encouraging me to join in the program and for providing important guidance on how to approach trade publishing as an academic. My writing cohort, in particular Elaine Blacklock, Kate Burnham, Maryanna Gabriel, Cindy Littlefair, Martha Morrison, Jessica Payne, and Adelle Purdham, provided encouragement and support during the early drafting of various chapters. My MFA mentor, Jane Silcott, read almost all the manuscript and shared her exquisite talent for caressing language as she relentlessly urged me to exercise my creative nonfiction chops.

My academic expertise is in developmental social psychology. This background as well as the personal experiences recounted in this book fermented my interest in the topic of guilt. But to do the topic justice, I had to go well beyond my comfort zone is researching the full range of areas covered in this book. My work was made so much easier by having access to a range of wonderful people in my broader academic and intellectual community. Simon Gadbois gave valuable input on how to think about animal social relations. Shannon Peng reviewed and refined my understanding of guilt in collectivist societies. Jessica Borelli generously shared her scale for measuring work-family conflict. Erin Dempsey helped with the chapter on psychopathology. Nameera Akhtar, Christopher Austin, Fatemeh Keshvari, Barry Lesser, Megan Sponagle, and Alexander Treiger provided important guidance in how to tell the story of guilt in religion. Kim Brooks, Stephen Coughlan, and Jennifer Llewelyn of Dalhousie's Schulich School of Law provided invaluable expertise on understanding the law. I valued greatly stimulating discussions with many other colleagues and friends, notably Sheila Blair-Reid, Elizabeth Frank, and Talan İşcan. Stef Hartlin was in on this book project from the beginning, and I am grateful for her support and enthusiasm. I owe her credit for the slogan "making friends with guilt." She has been making my life easier and more fun with her graft and her inspiration for nearly twenty years. I have enjoyed an even longer and exceptionally fruitful intellectual collaboration with John Barresi. He has been the best intellectual sparring partner for all ideas, including many of those in this book. I thank them all for their generosity. Any mistakes, in time-honored fashion, remain mine.

A large group of students at Dalhousie have helped along the way, in particular I thank Swaha Bhowmick, Daphne Bolduc, Laura Coon, Robin Curtis, Mya Dockrill, Andronika Kelso, Mackenzie Moore, and Megan Sponagle. During the last few years, the many students in my third year Experimental Social Psychology class at Dalhousie University embraced the project and provided great stories of how guilt shows up in their lives.

My editors at Collins Canada, Julia McDowell, and BenBella Books, Leah Wilson, were in equal parts encouraging and critical and that, I think, is exactly what great editors should be. Lauren McKeon at Collins guided the book through to publication in the most sensitive yet efficient way. Stacey Cameron and Natalie Meditsky expertly shepherded the manuscript through copyediting and page proofing. It's been a real pleasure working with all of them. My agent, Kelly Bergh at Lucinda Literary, has been a cheerleader and sounding board throughout the project. I am delighted we were able to bring it to life together.

My wife, Shannon, was an immense stabilizing force as I worked on this manuscript for the best part of five years. She read various drafts of the manuscript and provided the kind of general reader feedback I needed. She also generously allowed me to tell her guilt stories when I didn't really have my own. It is wonderful to share the birth of this book with you.

Notes

Introduction: A Personal Experience of Guilt

1. "Guilt," *Cambridge Dictionary*, https://dictionary.cambridge.org/dictionary/english/guilt.
2. Ernest Kline, *A Comprehensive Etymological Dictionary of the English Language* (Amsterdam: Elsevier, 1971), 686.
3. "Guilt (emotion)," Wikipedia. The Free Encyclopedia, https://en.wikipedia.org/wiki/Guilt_(emotion), accessed June 30, 2023.
4. Roy Baumeister et al., "Guilt: An Interpersonal Approach," *Psychological Bulletin* 115, no. 2 (1994), 243–267.

Chapter one: What Is Guilt?

1. Sigmund Freud, "Civilization and Its Discontents," in *The Standard Edition of the Complete Works of Sigmund Freud*. Vol. 21, ed. James Strachey (New York: Norton, 1930/1961), 64–145.
2. Freud recognizes this as he writes in his final chapter, "Having reached the end of his journey, the author must ask his reader's forgiveness for not having been a more skilful guide and for not having spared them empty stretches of road and troublesome detours" (Freud, "Civilization and Its Discontents," 134).
3. "Civilization…obtains mastery over the individual's dangerous desire for aggression by weakening and disarming it and by setting up an agency [the superego] within him to watch over it, like a garrison in a conquered city" (Freud, "Civilization and Its Discontents," 123–124).
4. Yoel Inbar et al., "Moral Masochism: On the Connection between Guilt and Self-Punishment," *Emotion* 13, no. 1 (February 2013): 14–18, https://doi.org/10.1037/a0029749.

5. Freud, "Civilization and Its Discontents," 124 (my emphasis).
6. Freud, "Civilization and Its Discontents," 127.
7. See Colwyn Trevarthen, "Communication and Cooperation in Early Infancy: A Description of Primary Intersubjectivity," in *Before Speech: The Beginning of Human Communication*, ed. Margaret Bullowa, (London: Cambridge University Press, 1979), 321–347; T. Berry Brazelton et al., "The Origins of Reciprocity: The Early Mother-Infant Interaction," in *The Effect of the Infant on Its Caregiver*, ed. Michael Lewis and Leonard Rosenblum (New York: Wiley, 1974), 49–76.
8. Roy Baumeister et al., "Guilt: An Interpersonal Approach," *Psychological Bulletin* 115, no. 2 (1994): 243–267.
9. Baumeister et al., "Guilt," 245.
10. Baumeister et al., "Guilt," 246.
11. Paul Bloom, *Against Empathy: The Case for Rational Compassion* (Hopewell, NJ: Ecco Press, 2016).
12. Martin L. Hoffman, "Development of Prosocial Behavior: Empathy and Guilt," in *The Development of Social Behavior*, ed. Nancy Eisenberg (New York: Academic Press, 1982), 281–313.
13. Although Freud had focused on the internalized anger of guilt, the involvement in guilt of both self-directed anger and compassion for others was recognized by certain psychoanalytic theorists who followed Freud. For example, Melanie Klein distinguished between "persecutory guilt," which emphasizes anger toward the self and "reparative guilt," which emphasizes caring toward the other. See Donald L. Carveth, *Guilt: A Contemporary Introduction* (Abingdon, Oxon: Routledge, 2024).
14. Jerome H. Barkow, "Beneath New Culture Is Old Psychology: Gossip and Social Stratification," in *The Adapted Mind*, ed. Jerome H. Barkow et al. (New York: Oxford University Press, 1992), 627–638.
15. Maryam Kouchaki et al., "The Burden of Guilt: Heavy Backpacks, Light Snacks, and Enhanced Morality," *Journal of Experimental Psychology: General* 143, no. 1 (2014): 414–424, https://doi.org/10.1037/a0031769; Martin V. Day and D. Ramona Bobocel, "The Weight of a Guilty Conscience: Subjective Body Weight as

an Embodiment of Guilt," *PLOS One*, 8 (2013): 1–7, https://doi.org/10.1371/journal.pone.0069546.
16. The difference was first articulated clearly by Helen Lewis in 1971. See Helen Block Lewis, *Shame and Guilt in Neurosis* (New York: International Universities Press, 1971); see also June P. Tangney and Ronda L. Dearing, *Shame and Guilt* (New York: Guilford Press, 2001).
17. Alessio Nencini and Anna Maria Meneghini, "How Relational Bonds Influence Strategies for Coping with Guilt," *Journal of Relationships Research* 4, e9 (2013): 1–7, https://doi.org/10.1017/jrr.2013.9.
18. These two recipes roughly correspond to what psychoanalysts sometimes call "persecutory" and "reparative" guilt, see Carveth, *Guilt*, 2. The distinction has also been recognized by psychologists who have explored it cross-culturally (e.g., Johnny R. Fontaine et al., "Untying the Gordian Knot of Guilt and Shame: The Structure of Guilt and Shame Reactions Based on Situation and Person Variation in Belgium, Hungary, and Peru," *Journal of Cross-Cultural Psychology* 37, no. 3 (2006): 273–292) and in childhood (e.g., Carolyn Zahn-Waxler and Grazyna Kochanska, "The Origins of Guilt," in *Socioemotional Development*, ed. Ross Thompson (University of Nebraska Press, 1990), 183–258).

Chapter two: What Is Guilt For?

1. James Fisher and Robert A. Hinde, "The Opening of Milk Bottles by Birds," *British Birds* 42 (1949): 347–359.
2. For example, Robert A. Hinde et al., "Nature and Determinants of Preschoolers' Differential Behaviour to Adults and Peers," *British Journal of Developmental Psychology* 1, no.1 (1983): 3–19.
3. Nicholas K. Humphrey, "The Social Function of Intellect," In *Growing Points in Ethology*, ed. Patrick P.G. Bateson and Robert A. Hinde (Cambridge: Cambridge University Press, 1976), 303–317.
4. Michael R. Rose, "The Mental Arms Race Amplifier," *Human Ecology* 8, no. 3 (1980): 285–293.
5. Robert L. Trivers, "The Evolution of Reciprocal Altruism," *The Quarterly Review of Biology* 46, no. 1 (1971): 35–57.

6. Trivers, "The Evolution of Reciprocal Altruism," 46 (my emphasis).
7. Frans de Waal, *Chimpanzee Politics. Power and Sex Among Apes.* (London: Cape, 1982).
8. De Waal, *Chimpanzee Politics*, 92.
9. Filippo Aureli et al., "Conflict Resolution Following Aggression in Gregarious Animals: A Predictive Framework," *Animal Behaviour* 64, no. 3 (2002): 325–343.
10. Annemieke Cools et al., "Canine Reconciliation and Third-Party-Initiated Postconflict Affiliation: Do Peacemaking Social Mechanisms in Dogs Rival Those of Higher Primates?" *Ethology* 114 (2008): 53–63.
11. Jane Goodall, "Feeding Behaviour of Wild Chimpanzees: A Preliminary Report," *Symposia of the Zoological Society of London* 10 (1963): 39–48.
12. Christophe Boesch, "The Emergence of Cultures among Wild Chimpanzees," *Proceedings of the British Academy* 88 (1996): 251–268.
13. Joan B. Silk, "The Form and Function of Reconciliation in Primates," *Annual Review of Anthropology* 31, no. 1 (2002): 21–44, https://doi.org/10.1146/annurev.anthro.31.032902.101743.
14. Frans de Waal, *Peacemaking among Primates* (Cambridge, MA: Harvard University Press, 2009), 36–78.
15. Frans de Waal and Filippo Aureli, "Conflict Resolution and Distress Alleviation in Monkeys and Apes," Annals of the New York Academy of Sciences 807 (1997): 317–328.
16. Filippo Aureli et al., "Conflict Resolution Following Aggression in Gregarious Animals: A Predictive Framework," *Animal Behaviour* 64, no. 3 (September 2002): 325–343, https://doi.org/10.1006/anbe.2002.3071; Kate Arnold and Andrew Whiten, "Post-Conflict Behaviour of Wild Chimpanzees (Pan Troglodytes Schweinfurthii) in the Budongo Forest, Uganda," *Behaviour* 138, no. 5 (2001): 649–690, https://doi.org/10.1163/156853901316924520.
17. Sonja E. Koski et al., "Reconciliation, Relationship Quality, and Postconflict Anxiety: Testing the Integrated Hypothesis in Captive Chimpanzees," *American Journal*

of *Primatology* 69, no. 2 (December 4, 2006): 158–172, https://doi.org/10.1002/ajp.20338.
18. Frans de Waal, "Bonobo Sex and Society," *Scientific American* 272, no. 3 (1995): 82–88, https://doi.org/10.1038/scientificamerican0395-82.
19. De Waal, "Bonobo Sex and Society," 85.
20. James Serpell and Priscilla Barrett, *The Domestic Dog: Its Evolution, Behavior and Interactions with People* (Cambridge, United Kingdom: Cambridge University Press, 2017).
21. Simona Cafazzo et al., "Dominance Relationships in a Family Pack of Captive Arctic Wolves (*Canis lupus arctos*): The Influence of Competition for Food, Age and Sex," *PeerJ* 4 (2016): e2707, https://doi.org/10.7287/peerj.2707v0.1/reviews/2.
22. Giada Cordoni and Elisabetta Palagi, "Reconciliation in Wolves (*Canis lupus*): New Evidence for a Comparative Perspective," *Ethology* 114, no. 3 (2008): 298–308, https://doi.org/10.1111/j.1439-0310.2008.01474.x.
23. Paul H. Morris et al., "Secondary Emotions in Non-Primate Species? Behavioural Reports and Subjective Claims by Animal Owners," *Cognition and Emotion* 22, no. 1 (2008): 3–20, https://doi.org/10.1080/02699930701273716.
24. Konrad Lorenz, *Man Meets Dog* (London: Methuen, 1954).
25. Julie Hecht et al., "Behavioral Assessment and Owner Perceptions of Behaviors Associated with Guilt in Dogs," *Applied Animal Behaviour Science* 139, no. 1–2 (2012): 134–142, https://doi.org/10.1016/j.applanim.2012.02.015.
26. Alexandra Horowitz, "Disambiguating the 'Guilty Look': Salient Prompts to a Familiar Dog Behaviour," *Behavioural Processes* 81 (2009): 447–452, doi:10.1016/j.beproc.2009.03.014.
27. Aaron Lazare, *On Apology* (New York: Oxford University Press, 2004), 35.
28. Ryan Fehr et al., "The Road to Forgiveness: A Meta-Analytic Synthesis of Its Situational and Dispositional Correlates," *Psychological Bulletin* 136, no. 5 (2010): 894–914, https://doi.org/10.1037/a0019993.
29. Padraic Gibson, "What's the Difference between Anxiety and Fear?" *Psychology Today*, June 13, 2023,

https://www.psychologytoday.com/us/blog/escaping-our-mental-traps/202301/whats-the-difference-between-anxiety-and-fear.
30. Yohsuke Ohtsubo and Ayano Yagi, "Relationship Value Promotes Costly Apology-Making: Testing the Valuable Relationships Hypothesis from the Perpetrator's Perspective," *Evolution and Human Behavior* 36, no. 3 (2015): 232–239, https://doi.org/10.1016/j.evolhumbehav.2014.11.008.
31. Jeni L. Burnette et al., "Forgiveness Results from Integrating Information about Relationship Value and Exploitation Risk," *Personality and Social Psychology Bulletin* 38, no. 3 (2011): 345–356, https://doi.org/10.1177/0146167211424582.
32. Daniel E. Forster et al., "Experimental Evidence That Apologies Promote Forgiveness by Communicating Relationship Value," *Scientific Reports* 11, no. 1 (2021): 13107, https://doi.org/10.1038/s41598-021-92373-y.
33. Helen Block Lewis, *Shame and Guilt in Neurosis* (New York: International Universities Press, 1971).
34. June P. Tangney and Ronda L. Dearing, *Shame and Guilt* (New York: The Guilford Press, 2002).
35. See Lisa Feldman Barrett, *How Emotions Are Made* (New York: Houghton Mifflin Harcourt, 2017).
36. Karen Caplovitz Barrett, "A Functionalist Approach to Shame and Guilt," in *Self-Conscious Emotions: The Psychology of Shame, Guilt, Embarrassment, and Pride,* ed. June P. Tangney and Kurt W. Fischer (New York: Guilford Press, 1995), 25–63.

Chapter three: The Development of Guilt and Conscience in Children

1. Sigmund Freud, "Civilization and Its Discontents," in *The Standard Edition of the Complete Works of Sigmund Freud.* Vol. 21, ed. James Strachey (New York: Norton, 1930/1961), 64–145.
2. Patricia J. Bauer, "Amnesia, Infantile," in *Encyclopedia of Infant and Early Childhood Development,* ed. Marshall M. Haith and Janette B. Benson (Academic Press, 2008): 51–62, https://doi.org/10.1016/B978-012370877-9.00007-4; Chris Moore and Karen Lemmon, eds., *The Self in Time: Developmental Perspectives* (Mahwah: Lawrence Erlbaum Associates, 2001).

3. David P. Ausubel, "Relationships between Shame and Guilt in the Socializing Process," *Psychological Review* 62, no. 5 (1955): 379, https://doi.org/10.1037/h0042534.
4. Chris Moore, *The Development of Commonsense Psychology* (New York: Psychology Press, 2006).
5. Jean Piaget and Bärbel Inhelder, *The Psychology of the Child* (New York: Basic Books, 1972).
6. Chris Moore, "Understanding Self and Others in the Second Year," in *Socioemotional Development in the Toddler Years: Transitions and Transformations*, ed. Celia Brownell and Claire Kopp (New York: Guilford Press, 2007), 43–65.
7. Markus Paulus et al., "When Do Children Begin to Care for Others? The Ontogenetic Growth of Empathic Concern across the First Two Years of Life," *Cognitive Development* 70 (2024): 101439, https://doi.org/10.1016/j.cogdev.2024.101439.
8. Martin L. Hoffman, "Development of Prosocial Behavior: Empathy and Guilt," in *The Development of Social Behavior*, ed. Nancy Eisenberg (New York: Academic Press, 1982), 281–313.
9. Pamela M. Cole et al., "Emotion Displays in Two-Year-Olds During Mishaps," *Child Development* 63, no. 2 (1992), 314–324, https://doi.org/10.1111/j.1467-8624.1992.tb01629.x.
10. Amrisha Vaish et al., "The Early Emergence of Guilt-Motivated Prosocial Behavior," *Child Development* 87, no. 6 (2016): 1772–1782, https://doi.org/10.1111/cdev.12628.
11. Grazyna Kochanska et al., "Guilt in Young Children: Development, Determinants, and Relations with a Broader System of Standards," *Child Development* 73, no. 2 (2002): 461–482, https://doi.org/10.1111/1467-8624.00418.
12. Grazyna Kochanska, "Socialization and Temperament in the Development of Guilt and Conscience," *Child Development* 62, no. 6 (1991): 1379–1392, https://doi.org/10.2307/1130813; Ross A. Thompson and Martin L. Hoffman, "Empathy and the Development of Guilt in Children," *Developmental Psychology* 16, no. 2 (1980): 155–156, https://doi.org/10.1037//0012-1649.16.2.155.
13. Karen Caplovitz Barrett et al., "Avoiders vs. Amenders: Implications for the Investigation of Guilt and Shame during Toddler-

hood?" *Cognition and Emotion* 7, no. 6 (1993): 481–505, https://doi.org/10.1080/02699939308409201.

14. Grazyna Kochanska et al., "Guilt in Young Children: Development, Determinants, and Relations with a Broader System of Standards," *Child Development* 73, no. 2 (2002): 461–482, https://doi.org/10.1111/1467-8624.00418.

15. Cheryl Minton et al., "Maternal Control and Obedience in the Two-Year-Old," *Child Development* 42, no. 6 (1971): 1873–1894, https://doi.org/10.2307/1127592.

16. See "Attachment," Psychology Today, accessed July 24, 2024, https://www.psychologytoday.com/ca/basics/attachment.

17. John Bowlby, *Attachment and Loss* (London: Hogarth Press; Institute of Psycho-Analysis, 1969).

18. Mary Ainsworth et al., *Patterns of Attachment: A Psychological Study of the Strange Situation.* (Hillsdale: Lawrence Erlbaum Associates, 1978).

19. The original Ainsworth study and the many studies that have followed it have found that most infants fit the secure pattern (usually around 55–60 percent) with a minority of infants divided among the insecure patterns. Stressful conditions such as very low socio-economic circumstances or having a single, adolescent mother tend to increase the likelihood of insecure attachment. See Sheri Madigan et al. "The First 20,000 Strange Situation Procedures: A Meta-Analytic Review," *Psychological Bulletin* 149, no. 1–2 (2023): 99–132.

20. Grazyna Kochanska, "Committed Compliance, Moral Self, and Internalization: A Mediational Model," *Developmental Psychology* 38, no. 3 (2002): 339–351, https://doi.org/10.1037//0012-1649.38.3.339; Marianne S. de Wolff and Marinus H. van IJzendoorn, "Sensitivity and Attachment: A Meta-Analysis on Parental Antecedents of Infant Attachment," *Child Development* 68, no. 4 (1997): 571–591, https://doi.org/10.2307/1132107.

21. Grazyna Kochanska and Nazan Aksan, "Children's Conscience and Self-Regulation," *Journal of Personality* 74, no. 6 (2006): 1587–1618, https://doi.org/10.1111/j.1467-6494.2006.00421.x.

22. Martin L. Hoffman, "Childrearing Practices and Moral Development: Generalizations from Empirical

Research," *Child Development* 34, no. 2 (1963): 295–318, https://doi.org/10.2307/1126729.
23. Grazyna Kochanska, "Socialization and Temperament in the Development of Guilt and Conscience," *Child Development* 62, no. 6 (1991): 1379–1392, https://doi.org/10.2307/1130813.
24. Donald L. Carveth, *Guilt: A Contemporary Introduction* (Abingdon, Oxon: Routledge, 2024).
25. Kochanska, "Socialization and Temperament."
26. Erika Baker et al., "Development of Fear and Guilt in Young Children: Stability over Time and Relations with Psychopathology," *Development and Psychopathology* 24, no. 3 (2012): 833–845, https://doi.org/10.1017/s0954579412000399.
27. Kochanska, "Socialization and Temperament."

Chapter four: Guilt-Proneness

1. Ray Cavanaugh, "What Lies Beneath: 80 Years of *The Mask of Sanity*," *The Lancet Psychiatry* 8, no. 11 (2021): 952–954, https://doi.org/10.1016/s2215-0366(21)00406-5.
2. Hervey M. Cleckley, *The Mask of Sanity: An Attempt to Clarify Some Issues about the So-Called Psychopathic Personality* (St Louis: Mosby, 1941).
3. The fifth edition of Cleckley's book is available in full on the internet. See Cleckley, *The Mask of Sanity*, https://www.gwern.net/docs/psychology/1941-cleckley-maskofsanity.pdf. I especially recommend reading the fifteen case histories to get a vivid picture of the lives of psychopaths.
4. The original Hare Psychopathy Checklist is available on the internet at Psychology Tools, https://psychology-tools.com/test/pcl-22.
5. Robert D. Hare, *Without Conscience: The Disturbing World of the Psychopaths among Us* (New York: Guilford Press, 1999).
6. John Archer, "Sex Differences in Aggression in Real-World Settings: A Meta-Analytic Review," *Review of General Psychology* 8, no. 4 (2004): 291–322, https://doi.org/10.1037/1089-2680.8.4.291; Kaj Björkqvist and Karin Österman, "Sex Differences in Aggression," in *The Routledge International Handbook of*

Human Aggression, ed. Jane Ireland et al. (London: Routledge, 2018), 47–58, https://doi.org/10.4324/9781315618777-2.
7. M.E. Thomas, Confessions of a Sociopath: A Life Spent Hiding in Plain Sight (New York: Crown, 2013). You can watch her describe her life experience in a series of videos at the Society for the Prevention of Disorders of Aggression YouTube site: https://www.youtube.com/@psychopathyis3353/videos.
8. M.E. Thomas, Confessions of a Sociopath, 16.
9. June P. Tangney and Ronda L. Dearing, Shame and Guilt (New York: The Guilford Press, 2002).
10. Jana L. Mullins-Nelson et al., "Psychopathy, Empathy, and Perspective-Taking Ability in a Community Sample: Implications for the Successful Psychopathy Concept," International Journal of Forensic Mental Health 5, no. 2 (2006): 133–149, https://doi.org/10.1080/14999013.2006.10471238.
11. For a quick introduction to the "Big Five" factor model of personality, see "Big 5 Personality Traits," Psychology Today, accessed June 6, 2023, https://www.psychologytoday.com/ca/basics/big-5-personality-traits.
12. Eileen K. Graham et al., "Trajectories of Big Five Personality Traits: A Coordinated Analysis of 16 Longitudinal Samples," European Journal of Personality 34, no. 3 (2020): 301–321. https://doi.org/10.1002/per.2259.
13. Susan Cain, Quiet: The Power of Introverts in a World That Can't Stop Talking (New York: Broadway Books, 2013).
14. Danielle Einstein and Kevin Lanning, "Shame, Guilt, Ego Development and the Five-Factor Model of Personality," Journal of Personality 66, no. 4 (1998): 555–582, https://doi.org/10.1111/1467-6494.00024.
15. Jo Ann Abe, "Shame, Guilt, and Personality Judgment," Journal of Research in Personality 38, no. 2 (2004): 85–104, https://doi.org/10.1016/s0092-6566(03)00055-2; Seval Erden and Müge Akbağ, "How Do Personality Traits Effect Shame and Guilt? An Evaluation of the Turkish Culture," Eurasian Journal of Educational Research 58 (2015): 113–132, https://doi.org/10.14689/ejer.2015.58.4; Peter Muris et al.,

"Shame on Me! Self-Conscious Emotions and Big Five Personality Traits and Their Relations to Anxiety Disorders Symptoms in Young, Non-Clinical Adolescents," *Child Psychiatry and Human Development* 49, no. 2 (2018): 268–278, https://doi.org/10.1007/s10578-017-0747-7.

16. Abe, "Shame, Guilt, and Personality Judgment," 85–104.
17. Ronald C. Johnson et al., "Guilt, Shame, and Adjustment in Three Cultures," *Personality and Individual Differences* 8, no. 3 (1987): 357–364, https://doi.org/10.1016/0191-8869(87)90036-5.
18. Jennifer V. Fayard et al., "Uncovering the Affective Core of Conscientiousness: The Role of Self-Conscious Emotions," *Journal of Personality* 80, no. 1 (2012): 1–32, https://doi.org/10.1111/j.1467-6494.2011.00720.x.
19. Nicole Else-Quest et al., "Gender Differences in Self-Conscious Emotional Experience: A Meta-Analysis," *Psychological Bulletin* 138, no. 5 (2012): 947–981. https://doi.org/10.1037/a0027930.
20. Tamas David-Barrett et al., "Women Favour Dyadic Relationships, but Men Prefer Clubs: Cross-Cultural Evidence from Social Networking," *PLOS ONE* 10, no. 3 (2015): e0118329, https://doi.org/10.1371/journal.pone.0118329.
21. Eiluned Pearce et al., "Sex Differences in Intimacy Levels in Best Friendships and Romantic Partnerships," *Adaptive Human Behavior and Physiology* 7, no. 1 (2020): 1–16, https://doi.org/10.1007/s40750-020-00155-z.
22. Jamie L. Walter and Stacey M. Burnaford, "Developmental Changes in Adolescents' Guilt and Shame: The Role of Family Climate and Gender," *North American Journal of Psychology* 8, no. 2 (2006): 321–338.
23. Cesar J. Rebellon et al., "The Relationship between Gender and Delinquency: Assessing the Mediating Role of Anticipated Guilt," *Journal of Criminal Justice* 44 (2016): 77–88, https://doi.org/10.1016/j.jcrimjus.2015.11.006.
24. Arne De Boeck et al., "The Social Origins of Gender Differences in Anticipated Feelings of Guilt and Shame Following Delinquency," *Criminology and Criminal Justice* 18, no. 3 (2017): 291–313, https://doi.org/10.1177/1748895817721273.

25. June P. Tangney and Ronda L. Dearing, *Shame and Guilt* (New York: The Guilford Press, 2002).
26. Ruth Benedict, *The Chrysanthemum and the Sword: Patterns of Japanese Culture* (Boston: Houghton Mifflin Co. 1946).
27. Geert Hofstede, *Culture's Consequences: International Differences in Work-Related Values* (Beverly Hills: Sage 1980).
28. Ying Wong and Jeanne Tsai, "Cultural Models of Shame and Guilt," in *The Self-Conscious Emotions: Theory and Research*, ed. June P. Tangney et al. (New York: The Guilford Press 2007), 209–223.
29. Sana Sheikh, "Cultural Variations in Shame's Responses," *Personality and Social Psychology Review* 18, no. 4 (2014): 387–403, https://doi.org/10.1177/1088868314540810.
30. Ying Wong and Jeanne Tsai, "Cultural Models of Shame and Guilt."
31. Charissa Cheah et al., "Confirming the Multidimensionality of Psychologically Controlling Parenting among Chinese-American Mothers: Love Withdrawal, Guilt Induction, and Shaming." *International Journal of Behavioral Development* 38 no. 3 (2015): 285–292, https://doi.org/10.1177/0165025414562238.
32. Quoted in Ying Wong and Jeanne Tsai, "Cultural Models of Shame and Guilt," 209.
33. Olwen Bedford and Kwang-Kuo Hwang, "Guilt and Shame in Chinese Culture: A Cross-Cultural Framework from the Perspective of Morality and Identity," *Journal for the Theory of Social Behaviour* 33, no. 2 (2003): 127–144, https://doi.org/10.1111/1468-5914.00210.
34. Bernard Williams, *Shame and Necessity* (Berkeley: University of California Press, 1993).
35. David Brooks "The Shame Culture," *The New York Times*, March 16, 2016, https://www.nytimes.com/2016/03/15/opinion/the-shame-culture.html: "The guilt culture could be harsh, but at least you could hate the sin and still love the sinner. The modern shame culture allegedly values inclusion and tolerance, but it can be strangely unmerciful to those who disagree and to those who don't fit in."

Notes

Chapter five: Guilt in Adult Relationships

1. Infidelity is conservatively estimated to occur in 25 percent of North American marriages. It is likely much higher in less committed romantic relationships. See Frank D. Fincham and Ross W. May, "Infidelity in Romantic Relationships," *Current Opinion in Psychology* 13 (2017): 70–74, https://doi.org/10.1016/j.copsyc.2016.03.008.
2. Roy Baumeister et al., "Personal Narratives about Guilt: Role in Action Control and Interpersonal Relationships," *Basic and Applied Social Psychology* 17, no. 1 (1995): 173–198, https://doi.org/10.1207/s15324834basp1701&2_10.
3. Margaret S. Clark and Judson Mills, "Interpersonal Attraction in Exchange and Communal Relationships," *Journal of Personality and Social Psychology* 37, no. 1 (1979): 12–24, https://doi.org/10.1037//0022-3514.37.1.12.
4. Margaret S. Clark and Judson R. Mills, "A Theory of Communal (and Exchange) Relationships," in *Handbook of Theories of Social Psychology*, ed. Paul A.M. Van Lange et al. (Thousand Oaks: Sage Publications Ltd., 2012), 232–250, https://doi.org/10.4135/9781446249222.n38.
5. You can try them out here: "Clark Relationship Science Laboratory at Yale University /Scales and Measures," https://clarkrelationshiplab.yale.edu/scales-and-measures.
6. Margaret S. Clark et al., "Recipient's Mood, Relationship Type, and Helping," *Journal of Personality and Social Psychology* 53, no. 1 (1987): 94–103, https://doi.org/10.1037//0022-3514.53.1.94.
7. Laura Coon, "It's Not You, It's Me: Individual Factors Associated with Attachment and Relationship Satisfaction" (M.Sc. thesis, Dalhousie University, 2023), https://dalspace.library.dal.ca/items/367a7194-b5b1-444e-a567-5d6ca1c2fa6d.
8. Robin Dunbar, *Friends: Understanding the Power of Our Most Important Relationships* (London: Abacus, 2021).
9. Kristin Gustavson et al., "Life Satisfaction in Close Relationships: Findings from a Longitudinal Study," *Journal of Happiness Studies* 17, no. 3 (2015): 1293–1311, https://doi.org/10.1007/s10902-015-9643-7.

10. Nancy K. Grote and Margaret S. Clark, "Distributive Justice Norms and Family Work: What Is Perceived as Ideal, What Is Applied, and What Predicts Perceived Fairness?" *Social Justice Research*, 1998, 243–269.
11. Sigmund Freud, "Three Essays on the Theory of Sexuality," in *The Standard Edition of the Complete Works of Sigmund Freud*. Vol.7, ed. James Strachey (New York: Norton, 1905/1949), 135–245.
12. John Bowlby, *Attachment and Loss* (London: Hogarth Press; Institute of Psycho-Analysis, 1969).
13. Cindy Hazan and Phillip Shaver, "Romantic Love Conceptualized as an Attachment Process," *Journal of Personality and Social Psychology* 52, no. 3 (1987): 511–524, https://doi.org/10.1037//0022-3514.52.3.511.
14. Ashley S. Holland et al., "Attachment Styles in Dating Couples: Predicting Relationship Functioning over Time," *Personal Relationships* 19, no. 2 (2012): 234–246, https://doi.org/10.1111/j.1475-6811.2011.01350.x; Octav-Sorin Candel and Maria Nicoleta Turliuc, "Insecure Attachment and Relationship Satisfaction: A Meta-Analysis of Actor and Partner Associations," *Personality and Individual Differences* 147 (2019): 190–199, https://doi.org/10.1016/j.paid.2019.04.037.
15. Frederick G. Lopez et al., "Attachment Styles, Shame, Guilt, and Collaborative Problem-Solving Orientations," *Personal Relationships* 4, no. 2 (1997): 187–199, https://doi.org/10.1111/j.1475-6811.1997.tb00138.x.
16. June P. Tangney et al., "Test of Self-Conscious Affect–3," *PsycTESTS Dataset*, 2000, https://doi.org/10.1037/t06464-000.
17. Kelly A. Brennan et al., "Self-Report Measurement of Adult Attachment: An Integrative Overview," in *Attachment Theory and Close Relationships*, ed. Jeffry A. Simpson and W. Steven Rholes (New York: The Guilford Press, 1998), 46–76.
18. Jennifer A. Bartz and John E. Lydon, "Navigating the Interdependence Dilemma: Attachment Goals and the Use of Communal Norms with Potential Close Others," *Journal of Personality and Social Psychology* 91, no. 1 (2006): 77–96, https://doi.org/10.1037/0022-3514.91.1.77.

19. Carolyn Birnie et al., "Attachment Avoidance and Commitment Aversion: A Script for Relationship Failure," *Personal Relationships* 16, no. 1 (2009): 79–97, https://doi.org/10.1111/j.1475-6811.2009.01211.x; C. Nathan DeWall et al., "So Far Away from One's Partner, Yet So Close to Romantic Alternatives: Avoidant Attachment, Interest in Alternatives, and Infidelity," *Journal of Personality and Social Psychology* 101, no. 6 (2011): 1302–1316, https://doi.org/10.1037/a0025497.
20. Marisa G. Franco, *Platonic: How the Science of Attachment Can Help You Make—and Keep—Friends* (New York: G. P. Putnam's Sons, 2022).
21. Danu A. Stinson et al., "The Friends-to-Lovers Pathway to Romance: Prevalent, Preferred, and Overlooked by Science," *Social Psychological and Personality Science* 13, no. 2 (2022): 562–571, https//doi.org/10.1177/9485506211026992.
22. Dunbar, *Friends*, 26.
23. Robin Dunbar, "Dunbar's Number: Why My Theory That Humans Can Only Maintain 150 Friendships Has Withstood 30 Years of Scrutiny" *The Conversation*, May 12, 2021, https://theconversation.com/dunbars-number-why-my-theory-that-humans-can-only-maintain-150-friendships-has-withstood-30-years-of-scrutiny-160676.
24. Dunbar, *Friends*, 32–33.
25. Dunbar, *Friends*, 43.
26. Marie G. Oldeman et al., "Friendships in Emerging Adulthood: The Role of Parental and Friendship Attachment Representations and Intimacy," *Personality and Social Psychology Bulletin* 51, no. 4 (2025): 514–529, https://doi.org/10.1177/01461672231195339.
27. Savannah Boele et al., "Linking Parent-Child and Peer Relationship Quality to Empathy in Adolescence: A Multilevel Meta-Analysis," *Journal of Youth and Adolescence* 48, no. 6 (2019): 1033–1055, https://doi.org/10.1007/s10964-019-00993-5.
28. David M. Levy, "Sibling Rivalry Studies in Children of Primitive Groups," *American Journal of Orthopsychiatry* 9, no. 1 (1939): 205–214, https://doi.org/10.1111/j.1939-0025.1939.tb05585.x.
29. Mike Fitz, "Siblicide: An Inextricable Behavior in Birds?" Explore Blog, April 26, 2022,

https://blog.explore.org/siblicide-an-inextricable-behavior-in-birds/.
30. Dieter Wolke and Slava Dantchev, "Sibling Bullying," in *The Wiley Blackwell Handbook of Bullying: A Comprehensive and International Review of Research and Intervention*, ed. Peter K. Smith and James O'Higgins Norman (New York: Wiley, 2021), 94–125.
31. "Sibling Bullying: 'I Wished I Hadn't Been Born,'" BBC News, November 13, 2013, https://www.bbc.com/news/magazine-24867267.
32. Judy Dunn and Carol Kendrick, *Siblings: Love, Envy, and Understanding* (Cambridge: Harvard University Press, 1982).
33. Anita L. Vangelisti et al., "Making People Feel Guilty in Conversations: Techniques and Correlates," *Human Communication Research* 18, no. 1 (1991): 3–39, https://doi.org/10.1111/j.1468-2958.1991.tb00527.x.
34. Roy Baumeister et al., "Personal Narratives about Guilt: Role in Action Control and Interpersonal Relationships," *Basic and Applied Social Psychology* 17, no. 1 (1995): 173–198, https://doi.org/10.1207/s15324834basp1701&2_10.
35. Nickola C. Overall et al., "Attachment Anxiety and Reactions to Relationship Threat: The Benefits and Costs of Inducing Guilt in Romantic Partners," *Journal of Personality and Social Psychology* 106, no. 2 (2014): 235–256, https://doi.org/10.1037/a0034371.
36. Overall et al., "Attachment Anxiety and Reactions to Relationship Threat," 251.

Chapter six: Parental Guilt

1. At the time, we thought the nurse's "piranha" comment was an off-the-cuff joke. We only learned later that it is a common reference. See Elaine Burns, "'Like a Piranha': How Midwives' Descriptions of Breastfeeding Affect Women's Attitudes," The Conversation, February 28, 2024, https://the conversation.com/like-a-piranha-how-midwives-descriptions-of-breastfeeding-affect-womens-attitudes-48608.
2. Jessica Ashley, "'The First Time I Saw My Adopted Child,'" Mom.com, September 26, 2012, https://mom.com/kids/4142-first-time-i-saw-my-adopted-child.

3. In 2017, *Today's Parent* magazine declared screen time the number one source of "mom guilt" based on a survey of one thousand Canadian women. Jessica Spera, "This Is the #1 Source of Mom Guilt," *Today's Parent*, March 29, 2017, https://www.todaysparent.com/blogs/this-is-the-1-source-of-mom-guilt/.
4. Robert L. Trivers, "Parent-Offspring Conflict," *American Zoologist* 14, no. 1 (1974): 249–264, https://doi.org/10.1093/icb/14.1.249.
5. Robert Simmons, "Offspring Quality and the Evolution of Cainism," *Ibis* 130, no. 4 (1988): 339–357, https://doi.org/10.1111/j.1474-919x.1988.tb00992.x.
6. Claire Howorth, "The Goddess Myth: Why Many New Mothers Feel Guilt and Shame," *Time*, October 19, 2017, https://time.com/4989068/motherhood-is-hard-to-get-wrong/.
7. Yitzchak Ben Mocha et al. "What Is Cooperative Breeding in Mammals and Birds? Removing Definitional Barriers for Comparative Research," *Biological Reviews* 98 (2023), 1845–1861, https/doi.org/10.1111/brv.12986.
8. "Benefits of Breastfeeding," Cleveland Clinic, n.d., https://my.clevelandclinic.org/health/articles/15274-benefits-of-breastfeeding.
9. Judy Shakespeare et al., "Breast-Feeding Difficulties Experienced by Women Taking Part in a Qualitative Interview Study of Postnatal Depression," *Midwifery* 20 (2004): 251–260, https://doi.org/10.1016/j.midw.2003.12.011.
10. "Benefits of Breastfeeding," Cleveland Clinic.
11. Jessica L. Borelli et al., "Bringing Work Home: Gender and Parenting Correlates of Work-Family Guilt among Parents of Toddlers," *Journal of Child and Family Studies* 26, no. 6 (2017): 1734–1745, https://doi.org/10.1007/s10826 -017-0693-9.
12. Borelli et al. "Bringing Work Home," 1742.
13. Zeynep Aycan and Mehmet Eskin, "Relative Contributions of Childcare, Spousal Support, and Organizational Support in Reducing Work-Family Conflict for Men and Women: The Case of Turkey," *Sex Roles* 53, no. 7–8 (2005): 453–471, https://doi.org/10.1007/s11199-005-7134-8; Lianne Aarntzen

et al., "Work-Family Guilt as a Straightjacket. An Interview and Diary Study on Consequences of Mothers' Work-Family Guilt," *Journal of Vocational Behavior* 115 (2019): 103336, https://doi.org/10.1016/j.jvb.2019.103336.

14. Beth A. Livingston and Timothy A. Judge, "Emotional Responses to Work-Family Conflict: An Examination of Gender Role Orientation among Working Men and Women.," *Journal of Applied Psychology* 93, no. 1 (2008): 207–216, https://doi.org/10.1037/0021-9010.93.1.207; Pilar Martínez et al., "Family Gender Role and Guilt in Spanish Dual-Earner Families," *Sex Roles* 65, no. 11–12 (2011): 813–826, https://doi.org/10.1007/s11199-011-0031-4.

15. Claudia Goldin, "Excerpt from 'Career and Family' by Claudia Goldin," *Harvard Gazette*, October 17, 2023, https://news.harvard.edu/gazette/story/2023/10/excerpt-from-career-and-family-by-claudia-goldin/.

16. Lianne Aarntzen et al., "Work-Family Guilt as a Straightjacket."

17. Kendra Cherry, "Authoritative Parenting Characteristics and Effects," *Verywell Mind*, July 5, 2023, https://www.verywellmind.com/what-is-authoritative-parenting-2794956.

18. Jessica L. Borelli et al., "Bringing Work Home," 1743.

19. Bart Soenens, and Maarten Vansteenkiste, "A Theoretical Upgrade of the Concept Of Parental Psychological Control: Proposing New Insights on the Basis of Self-Determination Theory," *Developmental Review* 30, no. 1 (2010): 74–99, https://doi.org/10.1016/j.dr.2009.11.001.

20. Ortal Slobodin et al., "Mothers' Need Frustration and Controlling Parenting: The Moderating Role of Maternal Guilt," *Journal of Child and Family Studies* 29, no. 7 (2020): 1914–1926, https://doi.org/10.1007/s10826-020-01720-6.

21. Eunae Cho and Tammy D. Allen, "Relationship between Work Interference with Family and Parent-Child Interactive Behavior: Can Guilt Help?" *Journal of Vocational Behavior* 80, no. 2 (2012): 276–287, https://doi.org/10.1016/j.jvb.2011.12.002.

22. Laura Broadwell, "How Divorce Affects Children, Age by Age," *Parents Magazine*, September 6, 2023,

https://www.parents.com/parenting/divorce/coping/age-by-age-guide-to-what-children-understand-about-divorce/.

23. Matthijs Kalmijn, "Feelings of Guilt in the Family: The Case of Divorced Parents," in *Divorce in Europe: New Insights in Trends, Causes and Consequences of Relation Break-Ups*, ed. Dimitri Mortelman (Springer Nature, 2020), 271–289, https://doi.org/10.1007/978-3-030-25838-2_13.
24. Lori R. Kogan et al., "Disenfranchised Guilt—Pet Owners' Burden," *Animals* 12, no. 13 (2022), 1690, https://doi.org/10.3390/ani12131690.
25. Lori R. Kogan et al., "Dog Owners: Disenfranchised Guilt and Related Depression and Anxiety," *Human-Animal Interactions* 11, no. 1 (2023), https://doi.org/10.1079/hai.2023.0016.

Chapter seven: Guilt and Adult Children

1. Although there are not strict definitions, in Western cultures, the phase of adolescence usually covers the teen years, and the phase of emerging adult usually covers the years from late teens to mid-twenties. See Jeffrey J. Arnett, "Emerging Adulthood: A Theory of Development from the Late Teens through the Twenties," *American Psychologist* 55, no. 5 (2000): 469–480, https//doi.org/10.1037//0003-066X.55.5.469.066X.55.5.469.
2. Adam Shapiro, "Revisiting the Generation Gap: Exploring the Relationships of Parent/Adult-Child Dyads," *International Journal of Aging and Human Development* 58, no. 2 (2004):127–146.
3. German Posada and Ting Lu, "Child-Parent Attachment Relationships: A Lifespan Phenomenon," in *Handbook of Lifespan Development*, ed. Karen L. Fingerman et al. (New York: Springer, 2011), 87–115.
4. Kira S. Birditt et al., "Tensions in the Parent and Adult Child Relationship: Links to Solidarity and Ambivalence," *Psychology and Aging* 24, no. 2 (2009): 287–295, https//doi.org/10.1037/a0015196; Karen L. Fingerman, "Sources of Tension in the Aging Mother and Adult Daughter Relationship," *Psychology and Aging*, 11, no. 4 (1996): 591–606.

5. Victor G. Cicirelli, "Adult Children's Attachment and Helping Behavior to Elderly Parents: A Path Model," *Journal of Marriage and the Family* 45, no. 4 (1983): 815–825.
6. Daphna Oyserman et al., "Rethinking Individualism and Collectivism: Evaluation of Theoretical Assumptions and Meta-Analyses," *Psychological Bulletin* 128, no. 1 (2002): 3–72, https//doi.org/10.1037/0033-2909.128.1.3.
7. Gery C. Karantzas and Jeffry A. Simpson, "Attachment and Aged Care," in *Attachment Theory and Research: New Directions and Emerging Themes*, ed. Jeffry Simpson and Steven W. Rholes (New York: Guilford Press, 2015), 319–345.
8. Brian K. Barber et al., "Feeling Disrespected by Parents: Refining the Measurement and Understanding of Psychological Control," *Journal of Adolescence* 35, (2012): 273–287, doi:10.1016/j.adolescence.2011.10.010.
9. Brian K. Barber, "Psychological Control: Revisiting a Neglected Construct," *Child Development* 67, no. 6 (1996): 3296–3319.
10. Wendy M. Rote and Judith G. Smetana, "Situational and Structural Variation in Youth Perceptions of Maternal Guilt Induction," *Developmental Psychology* 53, no. 10 (2017): 1940–1953, http://dx.doi.org/10.1037/dev 0000396.
11. Duane Rudy et al., "Undergraduates' Perceptions of Parental Relationship-Oriented Guilt Induction Versus Harsh Psychological Control: Does Cultural Group Status Moderate Their Associations with Self-Esteem?" *Journal of Cross-Cultural Psychology* 45, no. 6 (2014): 905–920, https://doi.org/10.1177/0022022114532354.
12. Rin Reczek et al., "Parent–Adult Child Estrangement in the United States by Gender, Race/Ethnicity, and Sexuality," *Journal of Marriage and Family* 85, no. 2 (2023): 494–517, https://doi.org/10.1111/jomf.12898.
13. Forsaken_Stand_7503, "How to Deal with Estrangement Guilt?" https://www.reddit.com/r/EstrangedAdultChild/comments/-17xm6wo/how_to_deal_with_estrangement_guilt/?rdt=42534.
14. "Ageing and Health," World Health Organization, October 1, 2022, https://www.who.int/news-room/fact-sheets/detail/ageing-and-health.

15. GBD 2019 Dementia Forecasting Collaborators, "Estimation of the Global Prevalence of Dementia in 2019 and Prevalence in 2050: An Analysis for the Global Burden of Disease Study 2019," *Lancet Public Health* 7, (2022): e105–125, https://doi.org/https://doi.org/10.1016/S2468-2667(21)00249-8.
16. Richard Schulz et al. "Family Caregiving for Older Adults," *Annual Review of Psychology* 71, no. 1 (2020): 635–659, https//doi.org/10.1146/annurev-psych-010419-050754.
17. Mark J. Yaffe, "Implications of Caring for an Aging Parent," *Canadian Medical Association Journal* 138, no. 3 (1988): 231–235.
18. Andrés Losada et al., "Development and Validation of the Caregiver Guilt Questionnaire," *International Psychogeriatrics* 22, no. 4 (2010): 650–660, https://doi.org/10.1017/s1041610210000074; Louise Roach et al., "Validation of the Caregiver Guilt Questionnaire (CGQ) in a Sample of British Dementia Caregivers," *International Psychogeriatrics* 25, no. 12 (2013): 2001–2010, https://doi.org/10.1017/s1041610213001506; Laura Gallego-Alberto et al., "'I Feel Guilty'. Exploring Guilt-Related Dynamics in Family Caregivers of People with Dementia," *Clinical Gerontologist* 45, no. 5 (2022): 1294–1303, https://doi.org/10.1080/07317115.2020.1769244.
19. Dorothy A. Miller, "The 'Sandwich' Generation: Adult Children of the Aging," *Social Work* 26, no. 5 (1981): 419–423, https://doi.org/10.1093/sw/26.5.419.
20. Juliana Menasce Horowitz, "More than Half of Americans in Their 40s Are 'Sandwiched' Between an Aging Parent and Their Own Children," Pew Research Center, April 8, 2022, https://www.pewresearch.org/short-reads/2022/04/08/more-than-half-of-americans-in-their-40s-are-sandwiched-between-an-aging-parent-and-their-own-children/.
21. This and other comments from caregivers are taken from the qualitative study of caregiver's guilt in transitioning a loved one with dementia to a residential long-term care facility by Tamara L. Statz and her colleagues. See Tamara L. Statz et al., "'We Moved Her Too Soon': Navigating Guilt among Adult Child and Spousal Caregivers of Persons Living with Dementia Following a Move into Residential Long-Term Care," *Couple*

and *Family Psychology: Research and Practice* 11, no. 4 (2022): 300–314, https://doi.org/10.1037/cfp0000150.
22. Judith G. Gonyea et al., "Adult Daughters and Aging Mothers: The Role of Guilt in the Experience of Caregiver Burden," *Aging and Mental Health* 12, no. 5 (2008): 559–567, https://doi.org/10.1080/13607860802343027.
23. Andrés Losada et al., "Ambivalence and Guilt Feelings: Two Relevant Variables for Understanding Caregivers' Depressive Symptomatology," *Clinical Psychology and Psychotherapy* 25, no. 1 (2018): 59–64, https://doi.org/10.1002/cpp.2116.
24. Matthijs Kalmijn, "Guilt in Adult Mother–Child Relationships: Connections to Intergenerational Ambivalence and Support," *Journals of Gerontology: Social Sciences* 75, no. 4, (2020): 879–888, https://doi.org/10.1093/geronb/gby077.
25. Andrés Losada et al., "Ambivalence and Guilt Feelings"; Andrés Losada-Baltar et al., "Longitudinal Effects of Ambivalent and Guilt Feelings on Dementia Family Caregivers' Depressive Symptoms," *Journal of the American Geriatrics Society* 72, no. 5 (2024): 1431–1441, https://doi.org/10.1111/jgs.18871.
26. Gery C. Karantzas and Jeffry A. Simpson, "Attachment and Aged Care," in *Attachment Theory and Research: New Directions and Emerging Themes*, ed. Jeffry A. Simpson and Steven W. Rholes (New York: The Guilford Press, 2015), 319–345.
27. German Posada and Ting Lu, "Child-Parent Attachment Relationships."
28. John Bowlby, *Attachment and Loss* (London: Hogarth Press; Institute of Psycho-Analysis, 1969/1982).
29. Caroline J. Browne and E. Shlosberg, "Attachment Theory, Ageing and Dementia: A Review of the Literature," *Aging and Mental Health* 10, no. 2 (2006): 134–142, https://doi.org/10.1080/13607860500312118; Bère M. Miesen, "Alzheimer's Disease, the Phenomenon of Parent Fixation and Bowlby's Attachment Theory," *International Journal of Geriatric Psychiatry* 8, no. 2 (1993): 147–153, https://doi.org/10.1002/gps.930080207.
30. Sharon M. Nelis et al., "Attachment in People with Dementia and Their Caregivers: A Systematic Review," *Dementia* 13, no. 6 (2013): 747–767, https://doi.org/10.1177/1471301213485232.

31. Carol Magai and Carl I. Cohen, "Attachment Style and Emotion Regulation in Dementia Patients and Their Relation to Caregiver Burden," *The Journals of Gerontology Series B: Psychological Sciences and Social Sciences* 53B, no. 3 (1998), P147-P154, https://doi.org/10.1093/geronb/53b.3.p147; Carol Magai et al., "Relation between Premorbid Personality and Patterns of Emotion Expression in Mid- to Late-Stage Dementia," *International Journal of Geriatric Psychiatry* 12, no. 11 (1997): 1092–1099.
32. Sonja Perren et al., "The Impact of Attachment on Dementia-Related Problem Behavior and Spousal Caregivers' Well-Being," *Attachment and Human Development* 9, no. 2 (2007): 163–178, https://doi.org/10.1080/14616730701349630; Dorothy Markiewicz et al., "An Exploration of Attachment Styles and Personality Traits in Caregiving for Dementia Patients," *The International Journal of Aging and Human Development* 45, no. 2 (1997): 111–132, https://doi.org/10.2190/t4q4-e8f0-jwt5-dbag.
33. Gery C. Karantzas and Jeffry A. Simpson, "Attachment and Aged Care."
34. Andrés Losada et al., "Ambivalence and Guilt Feelings."
35. Rosa Romero-Moreno et al., "Guilt Focused Intervention for Family Caregivers. Preliminary Results of a Randomized Clinical Trial," *Clinical Gerontologist* 45, no. 5 (2022): 1304–1316, https://doi.org/10.1080/07317115.2022.2048287.
36. Andrés Losada et al., "Ambivalence and Guilt Feelings."

Chapter eight: Guilt Gone Awry

1. See Allan Abbass, "Reaching Through Resistance: Advanced Psychotherapy Techniques," (Kensington: Seven Leaves Press, 2015).
2. Dorothy E. Stubbe, "The Therapeutic Alliance: The Fundamental Element of Psychotherapy," *Focus* 16, no. 4 (2018): 402–403, https://doi.org/10.1176/appi.focus.20180022.
3. Allan Abbass et al., (2012), "Intensive Short-Term Dynamic Psychotherapy: A Systematic Review and Meta-Analysis of Outcome Research," *Harvard Review of Psychiatry* 20, no. 2 (2012): 97–108, https://doi.org/10.3109/10673229.2012.677347.

4. For a detailed explanation of this emotional dynamic and the therapeutic process used in ISTDP to combat it, see Joel Town et al., "The Anger-Depression Mechanism in Dynamic Therapy: Experiencing Previously Avoided Anger Positively Predicts Reduction in Depression via Working Alliance and Insight," *Journal of Counselling Psychology* 69, no. 3 (2022): 326–336, https://doi.org/ 10.1037/cou0000581.
5. American Psychiatric Association, *Diagnostic and Statistical Manual of Mental Disorders, 5th edition, Text Revision*, (American Psychiatric Association Publishing, 2022).
6. Sangmoon Kim et al., "Shame, Guilt, and Depressive Symptoms: A Meta-Analytic Review," *Psychological Bulletin* 137, no. 1 (2011): 68–96, https://doi.org/ 10.1037/a0021466.
7. June P. Tangney et al., "Proneness to Shame, Proneness to Guilt, and Psychopathology," *Journal of Abnormal Psychology* 101, no. 3 (1992): 469–478. https://doi.org/10.1037//0021-843x.101.3.469.
8. Carlos Tilghman-Osborne et al., "Inappropriate and Excessive Guilt: Instrument Validation and Developmental Differences in Relation to Depression," *Journal of Abnormal Child Psychology* 40, no. 4 (2012): 607–620, https://doi.org/10.1007/s10802-011-9591-6.
9. Marcin Sekowski et al., "The Relations between Childhood Maltreatment, Shame, Guilt, Depression and Suicidal Ideation in Inpatient Adolescents," *Journal of Affective Disorders* 276, (2020): 667–677, https://doi.org/10.1016/j.jad.2020.07.056.
10. "What is Cognitive Behavioral Therapy?" American Psychological Association, https://www.apa.org/ptsd-guideline/patients-and-families/cognitive-behavioral.
11. "Eating Disorders," National Institutes of Mental Health, https://www.nimh.nih.gov/health/topics/eating-disorders.
12. Emily S. Frank, "Shame and Guilt in Eating Disorders," *American Journal of Orthopsychiatry* 61, no. 2 (1991): 303–306.
13. John Burney and Harvey J. Irwin, "Shame and Guilt in Women with Eating-Disorder Symptomatology," *Journal of Clinical Psychology* 56, no. 1 (2000): 51–61; Jane Bybee et al., "Guilt, Guilt-Evoking Events, Depression, and Eating Disorders," *Current Psychology* 15, no. 2 (1996): 113–127; Jennifer

L. Sanftner et al., "The Relation of Guilt to Eating Disorder Symptomatology," *Journal of Social and Clinical Psychology* 14, no. 4, (1995): 315–324.

14. Michael P. Craven and Erin M. Fekete, "Weight-Related Shame and Guilt, Intuitive Eating, and Binge Eating in Female College Students," *Eating Behaviors* 33 (2019): 44–48, https://doi.org/10.1016/j.eatbeh.2019.03.002.
15. "Eating Disorders," National Institute of Mental Health, https://www.nimh.nih.gov/health/topics/eating-disorders.
16. Hilde Bruch, *The Golden Cage: The Enigma of Anorexia Nervosa* (Cambridge: Harvard University Press, 1978).
17. Bruch, *The Golden Cage*, 89.
18. Michael Friedman, "Survivor Guilt in the Pathogenesis of Anorexia Nervosa," *Psychiatry* 48, no. 1 (1985), 25–39.
19. Friedman, "Survivor Guilt," 29–30.
20. While the family systems approach to treatment of anorexia nervosa is broadly supported, the condition can be resistant to therapy. In such cases, biological treatments including drugs and neuromodulation techniques such as deep brain stimulation may be explored. See Alexandra F. Muratore and Evelyn Attia, "Current Therapeutic Approaches to Anorexia Nervosa: State of the Art," *Clinical Therapeutics* 43, no. 1 (2021): 85–94, https://doi.org/10.1016/j.clinthera.2020.11.006.
21. American Psychiatric Association, *Diagnostic and Statistical Manual of Mental Disorders*.
22. William G. Niederland, "Psychiatric Disorders among Persecution Victims: A Contribution to the Understanding of Concentration Camp Pathology and Its After-Effects," *The Journal of Nervous and Mental Disease* 139 (1964): 458–474.
23. Niederland, "Psychiatric Disorders," 469.
24. Hillel Glover, "Survival Guilt and the Vietnam Veteran," *The Journal of Nervous and Mental Disease* 172, no. 7 (1988): 393–397.
25. Herbert Hendin and Anne Haas, "Suicide and Guilt as Manifestations of PTSD in Vietnam Combat Veterans," *American Journal of Psychiatry* 148, no. 5 (1991): 586–591.
26. "Perpetrators of Sexual Violence Statistics," Rape, Abuse, and Incest National Network, https://rainn.org/statistics/perpetrators-sexual-violence.

27. Konstantin Bub and Miriam J.J. Lommen, "The Role of Guilt in Posttraumatic Stress Disorder," *European Journal of Psychotraumatology* 8, (2017): 1407202, https://doi.org/10.1080/20008198.2017.1407202.
28. "PTSD Treatment Basics," U.S. Department of Veteran Affairs National Center for PTSD, https://www.ptsd.va.gov/understand_tx/tx_basics.asp.
29. For example, Trauma-Informed Guilt Reduction Therapy. See Sonya Norman, "Trauma-Informed Guilt Reduction Therapy: Overview of the Treatment and Research," *Current Treatment Options in Psychiatry* 9, (2022): 115–125, https://doi.org/10.1007/s40501-022-00261-7.

Chapter nine: Guilt in Religion

1. "Catechism of the Catholic Church, II The Lord's Day," The Holy See, https://www.vatican.va/archive/ENG0015/__P7O.HTM.
2. "Catechism of the Catholic Church, IV The Gravity of Sin: Mortal and Venial Sins," The Holy See, https://www.vatican.va/archive/ENG0015/__P6C.HTM.
3. Bernard Schlink, *Guilt about the Past* (Toronto: Anansi Press, 2010), 62.
4. As I later learned, exposure to religious pluralism is one of the main factors contributing to the general increase in secularization in the West. See Isabella Kasselstrand et al., "Beyond Doubt: The Secularization of Society," (New York: New York University Press, 2023).
5. Herant Katchadourian, *Guilt: The Bite of Conscience* (Stanford: Stanford University Press, 2010).
6. This religious tradition is now sometimes called "ethical monotheism." See "Issues in Jewish Ethics: Ethical Monotheism," Jewish Virtual Library, https://www.jewishvirtuallibrary.org/ethical-monotheism.
7. "A Portrait of Jewish Americans," Pew Research Center, October 1, 2013, https://www.pewresearch.org/religion/2013/10/01/jewish-american-beliefs-attitudes-culture-survey/.

8. "The Global Religious Landscape," Pew Research Center, December 18, 2012, https://www.pewforum.org/2012/12/18/global-religious-landscape-exec/.
9. "Abraham Tested, Genesis 22:1-19 New King James Version" Bible Gateway, https://www.biblegateway.com/passage/?search=Genesis%2022%3A119&version=NKJV.
10. Reuven P. Bulka, "Guilt From, Guilt Towards" *Journal of Psychology and Judaism* 11, no. 2 (1987): 72–90.
11. Mark Zborowski and Elizabeth Herzog, *Life Is with People: The Culture of the Shtetl* (New York: International Universities Press, 1952).
12. Simon Dein, "The Origins of Jewish Guilt: Psychological, Theological, and Cultural Perspectives," *Journal of Spirituality in Mental Health* 15, (2013): 123–137, https://doi.org/10.1080/19349637.2012.737682.
13. See Elizabeth J. Albertsen et al., "Religion and Interpersonal Guilt: Variations across Ethnicity and Spirituality," *Mental Health, Religion, and Culture* 9, no. 1 (2006): 67–84, https://doi.org/ 10.1080/13694670500040484.
14. "Death in Adam, Life in Christ, Romans 5:12-21 New King James Version" Bible Gateway, https://www.biblegateway.com/passage/?search=Romans%205&version=NKJV.
15. Kelsey Peeples, "What is Original Sin for St Augustine?" *The Collector*, December 23, 2023, https://www.thecollector.com/st-augustine-original-sin/.
16. Edouard Roditi, "Guilt, Repentance, and Atonement," *European Judaism: A Journal for the New Europe* 13, no. 1 (1979): 17–19.
17. Bart D. Ehrman, *How Jesus Became God: The Exaltation of a Jewish Preacher from Galilee* (San Francisco: HarperOne, 2014).
18. Bahar Davary, "Forgiveness in Islam: Is it an Ultimate Reality?" *Ultimate Reality and Meaning* 27, no. 2 (2004): 127–141, https://doi.org/10.3138/uram.27.2.127.
19. Mujgan Inozu et al., "Why Are Religious Individuals More Obsessional? The Role of Mental Control Beliefs and Guilt in Muslims and Christians," *Journal of Behavior Therapy and Experimental Psychiatry* 43 (2012): 959–966, https://doi.org/10.1016/j.jbtep.2012.02.004; Patrick Luyten et

al., "The Relationship between Religiosity and Mental Health: Distinguishing between Shame and Guilt," *Mental Health, Religion, and Culture* 1, no. 2 (1998): 165–184. https//doi.org/10.1080/13674679808406507.
20. Pehr Granqvist, *Attachment in Religion and Spirituality: A Wider View* (New York: The Guilford Press, 2020).
21. Pehr Granqvist, *Attachment in Religion*, 59.
22. Jacob A. Arlow, "Guilt" in *20th Century Jewish Religious Thought*, ed. Arthur A. Cohen and Paul R. Mendes-Flohr, (Philadelphia: The Jewish Publication Society, 2009): 306.
23. See İdris Danışman, "A Theological Dialogue on The Notion of Conscience (Vicdân) in Christianity and Turkish Islamic Thought" *Dialog* 46, no. 1 (2023): 1–13, https://doi.org/10.47655/dialog.v46i1.779; Paul L. Heck, "Conscience across Cultures: The Case of Islam," *The Journal of Religion* 94, no. 3 (2014): 292–324; Gilbert S. Rosenthal, "Is the Concept of Conscience Found in Judaism?" *Conservative Judaism* 64, no. 2 (2013), 3–25, https://doi.org/10.1353/coj.2013.0000.
24. Helen Costigane, "A History of the Western Idea of Conscience," in *Conscience in World Religions*, ed. Jayne Hoose (Leominster: Gracewing, 1999), 3–20.
25. For example, "There Is no Compulsion in Religion," Surah Al-Baqarah 2:256, https://quran.com/en/al-baqarah/256.
26. "Genesis 18:25 New King James Version," Bible Gateway, https://www.biblegateway.com/passage/?search=-Genesis%2018%3A25-27&version=NKJV.
27. İdris Danışman, "A Theological Dialogue," 6.
28. Phil Zuckerman, "Why Nations Are Becoming More Secular," *Skeptic* (February 4, 2023), https://www.skeptic.com/reading_room/why-nations-are-becoming-more-secular/.

Chapter ten: Guilt in the Law

1. Meghan Grant, "Ex-University Student Acquitted in Naked, Magic Mushroom–Fuelled Attack on Professor," CBC News, March 3, 2020, https://www.cbc.ca/news/canada/calgary/magic-mushrooms-matthew-brown-assault-defence-verdict-1.5483053.

Notes

2. Meghan Grant, "'We Really Needed to Hear That': Man Who Beat Calgary Professor While High on Mushrooms Apologizes to Victim," CBC News, November 14, 2019, https://www.cbc.ca/news/canada/calgary/mount-royal-university-attack-professor-defence-mushrooms-trial-day-3-1.5359656.
3. Howard Zehr, *Changing Lenses: Restorative Justice in Our Times* (Harrisonburg: Herald Press, 1990/2015), 70.
4. Emily Sherwin, "Legal Taxonomy," *Legal Theory*, 15 (2009): 25–54, https://doi.org/10.1017/S1352325209090041.
5. "Criminal Law," Cornell Law School Legal Information Institute, https://www.law.cornell.edu/wex/criminal_law.
6. Government of Canada Justice Laws Website, https://laws-lois.justice.gc.ca/eng/acts/c-46/.
7. Government of Canada Justice Laws Website, https://laws-lois.justice.gc.ca/eng/acts/c-46/.
8. "There's no Place for the State in the Bedrooms of the Nation," CBC Archives https://www.cbc.ca/player/play/video/1.4715835.
9. The Criminal Code of Canada Section 19 explicitly recognizes that ignorance of the law cannot be used as a defense. See "Ignorance of the Law," Government of Canada Justice Laws Website, https://laws-lois.justice.gc.ca/eng/acts/c-46/section-19.html.
10. "Death Penalty: Facts and Figures," Amnesty International, May 24, 2022, https://amnesty.ca/features/death-penalty-facts-and-figures/.
11. Michelle Alexander, *The New Jim Crow: Mass Incarceration in the Age of Colorblindness* (New York: The New Press, 2010).
12. "Record Suspension Decisions and Clemency Recommendations," Government of Canada, January 24, 2022, https://www.canada.ca/en/parole-board/corporate/transparency/reporting-to-canadians/performance-monitoring -report/2018-2019/rs-dcr.html#rec.
13. A moving documentary film describing the case and its aftermath was released in 2015: *The Elmira Case*, directed by Jonathan Steckley (2015, Waterloo, Canada: Rosco Films).

14. Howard Zehr, *Changing Lenses*, 183.
15. Valerij Zisman, "Making Guilt Productive: The Case for Restorative Justice in Criminal Law," in *Guilt: A Force of Cultural Transformation*, ed. Katharina von Kellenbach and Matthias Buschmeier, (New York: Oxford University Press, 2022), 123–141, https://doi.org/10.1093/oso/9780197557433.003.0007.

Chapter eleven: Collective Guilt

1. You can watch a film of the event and Brandt's explanation here: "Willy Brandt's Historic Request for Forgiveness in Warsaw," Britannica, https://www.britannica.com/video/180273/Willy-Brandt-Poland-West-German-Treaty-of-1970.
2. Elazar Barkan, *The Guilt of Nations: Restitution and Negotiating Historical Injustice* (New York: Norton, 2000).
3. See "$70 Billion on, Claims Conf. Marks 60 Years of Reparations from Germany," *Jewish Journal*, July 12, 2012, https://jewishjournal.com/news/world wide/106077/. It should be noted that not all commentators accept that reparations have been paid in full. See, for example, Matthias Buschmeier, "The Absence of Productive Guilt in Shame and Disgrace. Misconceptions in and of German Memory Culture from 1945 to 2020," in *Guilt: A Force of Cultural Transformation*, ed. Katharina von Kellenbach and Matthias Buschmeier (New York: Oxford University Press, 2022), 323–349, https://doi.org/10.1093/oso/9780197557433.003.0017.
4. The English version of the essay is published as Carl G. Jung, "After the Catastrophe," in *Essays on Contemporary Events: The Psychology of Nazism* (Princeton: Princeton University Press, 1945/1989), 50–73.
5. Theodor Adorno with Jeffrey K. Olick and Andrew J. Perrin, *Guilt and Defense: On the Legacies of National Socialism in Postwar Germany* (Cambridge: Harvard University Press, 2010).
6. Lars Rensmann, "Collective Guilt, National Identity, and Political Processes in Contemporary Germany" in *Collective Guilt: International Perspectives*, ed. Nyla Branscombe and Bertjan Doosje (New York: Cambridge University Press, 2004), 169–189.
7. Yascha Mounk, *Stranger in My Own Country* (New York: Farrar, Straus, and Giroux, 2014), 110–111.

8. See "International Migration Policies: Data Booklet," United Nations, https://www.un.org/development/desa/pd/sites/-www.un.org.development.desa.pd/files/files/documents/2020-/Jan/un_2017_internationalmigrationpolicies_databooklet.pdf.
9. Michael L. Wilson et al., "Lethal Aggression in *Pan* Is Better Explained by Adaptive Strategies Than Human Impacts," *Nature* 513 (2014): 414–417, https://doi.org/10.1038/nature13727.
10. Becky Little, "How the Nazis Were Inspired by Jim Crow," *History*, August 4, 2023, https://www.history.com/news/how-the-nazis-were-inspired-by-jim-crow.
11. The Convention on the Prevention and Punishment of the Crime of Genocide (CPPCG), which came into force in 1951. Philippe Sands provides an insightful biographical account of the major players, including Raphael Lemkin, in the legal developments of this era in his book: Philippe Sands, *East West Street: On the Origins of "Genocide" and "Crimes Against Humanity"* (New York: Vintage, 2016).
12. See "Political Apologies," Institute for the Study of Human Rights, Columbia University, https://www.-humanrightscolumbia.org/ahda/political-apologies.
13. Bob Joseph, *21 Things You May Not Know about the Indian Act: Helping Canadians Make Reconciliation with Indigenous Peoples a Reality* (Port Coquitlam: Indigenous Relations Press, 2018).
14. The Final Report of the Truth and Reconciliation Commission of Canada Volume 1 (Montreal and Kingston: McGill-Queen's University Press, 2015), 159.
15. See "Constitution Act, 1982 Section 35," First Nations and Indigenous Studies, The University of British Columbia, https://indigenousfoundations.arts.ubc.ca/constitution_act_1982_section_35/.
16. "Indian Residential Schools Settlement Agreement," Government of Canada, https://www.rcaanc-cirnac.gc.ca/eng/1100100015576/1571581687074.
17. See "Truth and Reconciliation Commission of Canada," National Centre for Truth and Reconciliation, University of Manitoba, https://nctr.ca/about/history-of-the-trc/truth-and-reconciliation-commission-of-canada/.

18. "Truth and Reconciliation Commission Reports," National Centre for Truth and Reconciliation, University of Manitoba, https://nctr.ca/records/reports/#trc-reports.
19. "Statement by Honourable Murray Sinclair on the Pope's Apology," Last Real Indians, July 28, 2022, https://lastrealindians.com/news/2022/7/28/statement-by-honourable-murray-sinclair-on-the-popes-apology.
20. Shelby Steele, *The Content of Our Character: A New Vision of Race in America* (New York: HarperCollins, 1991), 77.
21. "'I Have a Dream' Speech," History, December 19, 2023, https://www.history.com/topics/black-history/i-have-a-dream-speech.
22. Mark Whitaker, *Saying It Loud: 1966—The Year Black Power Challenged the Civil Rights Movement* (New York: Simon and Schuster, 2023), 6.
23. Michelle Alexander, *The New Jim Crow: Mass Incarceration in the Age of Colorblindness* (New York: The New Press, 2010). See Leah Wang, "Updated Data and Charts: Incarceration Stats by Race, Ethnicity, and Gender for All 50 States and D.C.," Prison Policy Initiative, September 27, 2023, https://www.prisonpolicy.org/blog/2023/09/27/updated_race_data/.
24. Ta-Nehisi Coates, *Between the World and Me* (New York: One World, 2015).
25. Ibram X. Kendi, *How to Be an Antiracist* (New York: One World, 2019).
26. Ta-Nehisi Coates, "The Case for Reparations," *The Atlantic*, June 2014, https://www.theatlantic.com/magazine/archive/2014/06/the-case-for-reparations/361631/.
27. See Harald Schmidt et al., "Is It Lawful and Ethical to Prioritize Racial Minorities for COVID-19 Vaccines?" *Journal of the American Medical Association* 324, no. 20, (2020): 2023–2024, https://doi.org/10.1001/jama.2020.20571.
28. Shelby Steele, *White Guilt: How Blacks and Whites Together Destroyed the Promise of the Civil Rights Era* (New York: Harper Perennial, 2007).
29. John McWhorter, *Woke Racism: How a New Religion Has Betrayed Black America* (New York: Portfolio/Penguin, 2021).

30. Coleman Hughes, *The End of Race Politics: Arguments for a Colorblind America* (New York: Thesis, 2024).
31. I personally recommend the book by economist Glenn Loury, *The Anatomy of Racial Inequality* (Cambridge: Harvard University Press, 2002) for thoughtful discussion of some of the relevant issues.
32. Patrick R. Grzanka et al., "The White Racial Affect Scale (WRAS): A Measure of White Guilt, Shame, and Negation," *The Counseling Psychologist 48*, no. 1 (2020): 47–77.
33. See also Lisa B. Spanierman, "White Guilt in the Summer of Black Lives Matter," in *Guilt: A Force of Cultural Transformation*, ed. Katharina von Kellenbach and Matthias Buschmeier, (New York: Oxford University Press, 2022), 41–58.
34. Kendi, *How to Be an Antiracist*, 210 (my emphasis).
35. Shelby Steele, *Shame: How America's Past Sins Have Polarized Our Country* (New York: Basic Books, 2015), 3. See Whitaker, *Saying It Loud*, 187.
36. See Whitaker, *Saying It Loud*, 187.
37. See Bertjan Doosje et al., "Guilt by Association: When One's Group Has a Negative History," *Journal of Personality and Social Psychology 75*, no. 4 (1998): 872–886; Mark A. Ferguson and Nyla R. Branscombe, "The Social Psychology of Collective Guilt," in *Collective Emotions: Perspectives from Psychology, Philosophy, and Sociology*, ed. Christian von Scheve and Mikko Salmela (New York: Oxford University Press, 2014), 251–265; Janet K. Swim and Deborah L. Miller, "White Guilt: Its Antecedents and Consequences for Attitudes toward Affirmative Action," *Personality and Social Psychology Bulletin 25*, no. 4 (1999): 500–515, https://doi.org/10.1177/0146167 299025004008.
38. Brandon D. Dull et al., "Can White Guilt Motivate Action? The Role of Civic Beliefs," *Journal of Youth and Adolescence* 50 (2021): 1081–1097, https://doi.org/10.1007/s10964-021-01401-7.
39. "Remarks by President Biden on Protecting the Right to Vote," Policy, January 11, 2022, https://www.policymagazine.ca/remarks-by-president-biden-on-protecting-the-right-to-vote/.
40. Aarti Iyer et al., "White Guilt and Racial Compensation: The Benefits and Limits of Self-Focus," *Personality*

and Social Psychology Bulletin 29, no. 1 (2003):117–129, https://doi.org/10.1177/0146167202238377.

41. Iyer et al., "White Guilt and Racial Compensation"; Adam A. Powell et al., "Inequality as Ingroup Privilege or Outgroup Disadvantage: The Impact of Group Focus on Collective Guilt and Interracial Attitudes," *Personality and Social Psychology Bulletin* 31, no. 4 (2005): 508–521, https://doi.org/10.1177/0146167042717132005.
42. Sarah Fredericks, *Environmental Guilt and Shame: Signals of Individual and Collective Responsibility and the Need for Ritual Responses* (New York: Oxford University Press, 2021).
43. See "Survey Shows 'Green Guilt' Is Up among Americans," Call 2 Recycle: Leading the Charge for Recycling, April 19, 2012, https://www.call2recycle.org/2012-green-guilt-survey/ accessed on November 4, 2022.
44. See Caroline Hickman et al., "Climate Anxiety in Children and Young People and Their Beliefs about Government Responses to Climate Change: A Global Survey," *The Lancet Planetary Health* 5, no. 12 (2021), E863-E873, https://doi.org/10.1016/s2542-5196(21)00278-3; Janet K. Swim et al., "OK Boomer: A Decade of Generational Differences in Feelings about Climate Change," *Global Environmental Change* 73 (2022): 102479, https://doi.org/10.1016/j.gloenvcha.2022.102479.
45. Mark A. Ferguson and Nyla R. Branscombe, "Collective Guilt Mediates the Effect of Beliefs about Global Warming on Willingness to Engage in Mitigation Behavior," *Journal of Environmental Psychology* 30, no. 2 (2010): 135–142, https://doi.org/10.1016/j.jenvp.2009.11.010.
46. Rachel Carson, *Silent Spring* (Boston: Houghton Mifflin, 1962).
47. Emma Smith, "Rising Sea Levels Are Threatening Farmland, Towns and a Major Transportation Route along the Nova Scotia–New Brunswick Border," CBC News, April 22, 2021, https://newsinteractives.cbc.ca/longform/at-the-crossroads; "Climate Crossroads: When Could Nova Scotia Become an Island?" YouTube, n.d., https://www.youtube.com/watch?v=qWYwZ714Uvw.

48. See Aljosja Hooijer and Ronald Vernimmen, "Global LiDAR land elevation data reveal greatest sea-level rise vulnerability in the tropics," *Nature Communications* 12 (2021): 3592, https://doi.org/10.1038/s41467-021-23810-9.
49. Charlotte Alter et al., "TIME 2019 Person of the Year—Greta Thunberg," Time, https://time.com/person-of-the-year-2019-greta-thunberg/.
50. See, for example, Nathan J. Shipley and Carena J. van Riper, "Pride and Guilt Predict Pro-Environmental Behavior: A Meta-Analysis of Correlational and Experimental Evidence," *Journal of Environmental Psychology* 79 (2022): 101753, https://doi.org/10.1016/j.jenvp.2021.101753.
51. Ian Adams et al., "Experienced Guilt, but Not Pride, Mediates the Effect of Feedback on Pro-Environmental Behavior," *Journal of Environmental Psychology* 71 (2020): 101476, https://doi.org/10.1016/j.jenvp.2020.101476.
52. Matthew J. Kotchen "Offsetting Green Guilt," *Stanford Social Innovation Review* 7, no. 2 (Spring 2009): 26–31.
53. "Carbon Footprint Offset for Individuals," ClimeCo, https://carbonfund.org/carbon-offsets/.

Conclusion: Making Friends with Guilt

1. As I write this section, the movie *Inside Out* 2 has just been released. In the movie, several new emotions are introduced into the story, but notably, guilt and shame were excluded because they made the movie "too heavy" according to director Kelsey Mann. See Cameron Bonomolo, *Inside Out* 2 Cut New Emotions: "It Was Too Heavy," Comicbook, April 21, 2024, https://comicbook.com/movies/news/inside-out-2-deleted-new-emotions-shame-guilt/.